REIKI

Spirituality Guide To Find Balance and Increase your Positive Energy, Overcoming the Daily Stress and Depression

(Achieve higher consciousness, Increase vitality and Awaken Third Eye)

Penelope Prasad

Published by Rob Miles

Penelope Prasad

All Rights Reserved

Reiki: Spirituality Guide To Find Balance and Increase your Positive Energy, Overcoming the Daily Stress and Depression (Achieve higher consciousness, Increase vitality and Awaken Third Eye)

ISBN 978-1-989990-23-0

All rights reserved. No part of this guide may be reproduced in any form without permission in writing from the publisher except in the case of brief quotations embodied in critical articles or reviews.

Legal & Disclaimer

The information contained in this book is not designed to replace or take the place of any form of medicine or professional medical advice. The information in this book has been provided for educational and entertainment purposes only.

The information contained in this book has been compiled from sources deemed reliable, and it is accurate to the best of the Author's knowledge; however, the Author cannot guarantee its accuracy and validity and cannot be held liable for any errors or omissions. Changes are periodically made to this book. You must consult your doctor or get professional medical advice before using any of the suggested remedies, techniques, or information in this book.

Upon using the information contained in this book, you agree to hold harmless the Author from and against any damages, costs, and expenses, including any legal fees potentially resulting from the application of any of the information provided by this guide. This disclaimer applies to any damages or injury caused by the use and application, whether directly or indirectly, of any advice or information presented, whether for breach of contract, tort, negligence, personal injury, criminal intent, or under any other cause of action.

You agree to accept all risks of using the information presented inside this book. You need to consult a professional medical practitioner in order to ensure you are both able and healthy enough to participate in this program.

Table of Contents

INTRODUCTION 1

CHAPTER 1: WHAT IS REIKI? 7

CHAPTER 2: CHI, CHAKRAS, AND REIKI 25

CHAPTER 3: REIKI AND THE SCIENCE BEHIND IT 34

CHAPTER 4: AN OVERVIEW OF REIKI 40

CHAPTER 5: THE 21-DAY CLEANSING PROCESS OR REIKI.. 45

CHAPTER 6: CHAKRAS AND AURAS 52

CHAPTER 7: HISTORY OF REIKI 62

CHAPTER 8: MEDICAL CONCERNS 78

CHAPTER 9: SYMBOLS 81

CHAPTER 10: THE PRINCIPLES AND SYMBOLS USED IN REIKI 102

CHAPTER 11: WHAT ARE REIKI CHAKRAS? 109

CHAPTER 12: REIKI HAND POSITIONS AND SELF-HEALING 125

CHAPTER 13: VERDICT - REIKI ATTUNEMENTS/INITIATIONS 132

CHAPTER 14: HOW REIKI WORKS 141

CHAPTER 15: IMPROVE YOUR PHYSICAL HEALTH 154

CHAPTER 16: REIKI TREATMENTS 170

CONCLUSION.. 182

Introduction

Man has been healing others since the beginning of time, as there has been a healing agent available in the invisible realm the entire time. See, at the core of the universe everything is energy. This energy is extremely powerful and useful for humankind in a variety of ways.

Before we get into the depths of Reiki, let's look at Reiki through a practical, tangible example that you can experience right away.

The idea of Reiki is that all through the universe there is a vibration or a frequency that permeates all things, including the stars, planets, humans, animals, plants, rocks, and even the air and water. Liken it to the Force from Star Wars. Imagine that anything that makes you feel upset or stressed out as static or a disturbance in the energy flowing through your mind and body. This harmonic frequency of the universe is vibrating very fast and can cause any slower, unhealthy vibrations you are having to attune to it such an amazing power so that you can feel happy and healthy.

If you know how to attune yourself to that energy and allow it to flow through your mind and body, it can make the static that makes you unhappy or feeling stressed harmonize. Ultimately, if that contended with, your body can heal the way it is supposed to heal.

This is the essence of Reiki.

It isn't magical or mystical any more than your cell phone is magical or mystical. It might be mysterious to you right now but this is because you do not fully understand it yet. As your understanding grows, so will your ability to use it.

Gratitude is the way

What really gets Reiki energy flowing nicely is gratitude, as gratitude is the ultimate teacher of Reiki vibrations. Think of tuning in a radio station and the difference a minute change will cause in the radio frequency and how easily you can hear the music or the static between frequencies. If you can really tune into Reiki, you will find it much easier to manipulate this energy.

Most Reiki masters will tell you that Reiki is a benevolent 'love' energy. This is a wonderful way to describe it. It encompasses gratitude, love, happiness and joy – all positive emotions. A simple way to put yourself into this mindset is to think about a person you feel gratitude or thankfulness toward. He or she will be someone that has done or said something to help you or somehow conferred a benefit upon you. This will help you to begin thinking positively, which is necessary to begin feeling the Reiki energy flowing through you.

Let's perform a short exercise to let you feel what this energy is like when you concentrate and let it manifest. You will learn more about these steps later on in this book.

Take a deep breath in.

Breathe out.

Take another deep breath in.

And breathe out again.

Call to mind someone you are grateful toward.

◦ This is someone who has been very kind, loving and generous toward you.

Lift your hands in front of you, palm up and about chest or belly high.

Invite the essence or spirit of that person into your hands.

◦ Reflect upon that person and all that they mean to you.

◦ Consider how your hands feel as you are holding this person's essence in your hands.

- You may feel your hands beginning to tingle or getting warmer.

Did you feel your hands beginning to tingle? This is how you can really connect with the healing energy associated with Reiki. You may notice that when you are in that moment of gratitude that you cannot hold an angry feeling. Gratitude and anger cannot be held in the same place at the same time.

Envision the flow

Visualization is powerful. Go ahead and envision that there is white light in the universe that is flowing through you. Envision this power to enter the crown of your head, wash down the back of your neck, through your shoulders, upper arms, forearms and coming out and extending out through your hands.

By now you should be feeling a tingle and/or a warmth in your hands. Imagine your hands being able to harmonize with the things that you touch.

Move your hands to the sides of your face.

Feel the warmth entering your cheeks from your hands.

Know that this calm and restorative energy can flow through you and wash through your skin and out through your feet.

This is how you can connect to the energy that is Reiki. The following chapters will give you the information about Reiki and a more in-depth exploration into how you can experience the energy of Reiki to help you to relax, reduce your stress levels and increase your natural energy.

Chapter 1: What Is Reiki?

Reiki means **"universal energy for life."** Reiki is a natural healing system from Japan.

Ki' is the essential energy in and around any living thing. Reiki functions in its own way with this vital force, much like acupuncture, tai chi and yoga. During the treatment,' Ki' is directed to the client through the hands of the practitioner.

Reiki helps on all levels: psychological, physical, emotional and spiritual, restoring equilibrium, improving health and well-being.

Reiki can also support other conventional and complementary forms of treatment and can help to minimize the adverse effects of medicines or medical treatment.

Everyone can learn Reiki to use it quickly and easily for themselves and others.

There is no need for special skills or experience.

A Reiki Treatment

The patient remains fully dressed during a Reiki session as Reiki moves through clothes and even plaster castings. The customer usually lies on a couch, futon or sits on a chair when they find it uncomfortable to lie down.

The Reiki practitioner puts his hands strategically and in a number of non-intrusive positions around the body of the patient. Every hand is held for a few minutes. The entire person is being treated, not just isolated areas.

No massage or manipulation involves Reiki. It involves a gentle touch of healing.

Treatments can take from one hour to one half, depending on the needs of the customer.

Four (4) Consecutive Reiki Treatments

If you have a chronic condition, something that has developed over a long period of time, it often needs more than one treatment. Four consecutive Reiki treatments Treatment can be a very powerful way to receive Reiki healing every day over four consecutive days, since the energy can move deeper and deeper every day and often have very profound healing results. The first diagnosis is a profoundly calming and transformative experience. Some very deep healing often begins on day two and three and then day four can feel like the completion of the cycle.

When receiving four Reiki treatments, it's advisable to make space in your life and don't have many more plans during these four days to maximize the benefits of those treatments.

How does Reiki feel?

Every person experiences Reiki differently, depending on the individual needs of the person.

People often feel deeply relaxed and peaceful during a treatment. Sensations may include a sensation of warmth or heat, coolness or color or tingling. Sometimes, we can have a physical or emotional reaction, showing that the cure processes of the body work and balance is restored.

HISTORY OF REIKI

As it's now done in the United States, Reiki dates back to Mikao Usui's teachings in Japan in the early 1920's. Usui was a religious aspirant for a lifetime, a lay monk, wife and two children. Throughout Usui's period, various lines of Buddhist, Taoist, and Shinto rituals coexisted with Japanese culture and religion as dominant themes.

Usui's deep spiritual practices culminated in a profound manifestation which led to the Reiki practice. This was most probably achieved in 1922.

Over the last four years of Usui's life, he traveled extensively in Japan giving his spiritual teachings to during two thousand practitioners but only 16 as Reiki masters. One of Chujiro Hayashi's master students was a former naval officer. Hayashi and Usui sought to exclude healing practices from the wider array of teachings of Usui in order to spread them more broadly.

Hayashi opened a Reiki clinic with Usui's blessings in Tokyo where 16 practitioners were given pair therapy. Hawayo Takata, a Japanese-American first generation, came to Hayashi for medical treatment, including asthma. Takata's health was restored for months of treatment and she became a devoted student.

Takata introduced Reiki to Hawaii in 1937 and finally to the U.S. mainland with Hayashi's active guidance and support. 40 years before Takata started training Reiki

Masters (practitioners inspired to instruct others) she studied and taught Reiki. Her 22 Reiki specialist have spread her teachings since Takata's death in December 1980. However, Reiki has now become very popular and is now practiced worldwide, even though Takata is not generally taught in the traditional way.

HOW DOES REIKI WORKS?

At the easiest, most apparent point, Reiki therapy appears to help reduce stress, loosening pressure from the whole process. Not only does the individual move towards his or her unique balance of mind, body and spirit but also the body's own healing mechanisms often start to work more effectively depending on the level of physical health.

What Does Reiki Do?

How does Reiki relieve pressure and help the body recover exactly? This question also needs to be answered. While growing proof of Reiki's effects (for example, decreased heart rate, blood pressure, and stress hormones; improved immune strength) is being reported, we have only specific hypotheses on the cause of these effects or mechanisms of cure.

The complex process involving a number of body systems, simultaneously or in rapid succession, reverses the body from domination by the "fight-or-flight" anxiety response to the restoration response and support the body's own healing mechanisms. Many researchers theorize that the Reiki's physical, cognitive, emotional and spiritual healing impact is caused on a sub-physical level-perhaps in what science calls the bio-field. (See the Mind Body Therapies page for more information on the relaxation response)

What's the bio-field?

Bio-field is the term medical science used for the dynamic vibrational energy field, which is said to surround and penetrate the physical body. The bio-field is extremely subtle and no traditional scientific technology can yet document or study its existence directly. But traditional indigenous, pre-scientific medical systems have recognized a balanced and equally vibrant bio-field as the basis for health and wellbeing for thousands of years, and considered any disruption in the balance to be the beginning of disease.

By ritual drumming, instruments like the didgeridoo, tamboura and chant, over-toning and shrinking, the vibration is used in the healing rituals of indigenous cultures around the world. In addition, science is increasingly supporting the therapeutic value of vibration in the forms of sound and music. Perhaps Reiki's advantages come from the same vibratory mechanism, a process that probably involves increased coherence and decreasing system dissonance.

One theory is that the hands of the Reiki doer contain the energy vibrations of the wellness of the recipient. The outmost effect of Reiki could be perceived as a shift in awareness of the well-being that exists deep inside it independently of the current level of health. Reiki might then be understood to reincarnate the recipient in a process similar to the way that the grandfather clocks the same room to the rhythm of the dominant clock or how we relax if we are deeply peaceful in the presence of someone. Reiki seems to bind the practitioner with an internal sense of healing irrespective of how he or she is actually feeling.

Most treatments are aimed at restoring balance in bio-field acupuncture, qigong, shiatsu and pranayama. Reiki seems to be the most subtle one of these treatments and balances the recipient by subtle Reiki vibrations rather than by manipulation or even the gentlest force. It is also conceivable that Reiki, which some practitioners find more like therapy rather than energy therapies, does not come from the bio-field but comes from an even more elusive source: what physicists referred to as the unified field.

What Is The Relationship Between Reiki And Other Integrative Treatments?

Reiki is described by the National Center for Complementary and Integrative Health (NCCIH) as a complete alternative medical practice using supposed (although measured) energy fields or bio-fields that affect health. Energy-bio-field therapies "generally reflect the notion that human beings are infused with subtle energy sources," which believe in the human form and in the interpenetration. Energy treatments, such as therapeutic touch and healing touch, are thought to balance these subtle fields of energy.

Many Reiki practitioners consider Reiki different from other treatments and similar to meditation. While most energy therapies use methods to analyze the bio-field of the patient and make specific changes, Reiki practitioners do not prescribe and will not reorganize the bio-field purposely.

The nature of Reiki is extremely passive. The hands of the Reiki practitioner stay for most of the care and only move to switch hand positions. The Reiki doer is positive, he does not try to fix or alter the bio-field. In addition, the practitioner does not control Reiki energy in any way. She / he only sits lightly on the body (or just above the body in the presence of an open wound or burn, for example).

Reiki energy in the hands of the practitioner arises spontaneously in response to the need for balance for the individual beneficiary during that particular period. Each Reiki treatment is thus automatically tailored to that particular recipient's immediate need, even though the practitioner is allowed to use the same sequence of hand placements for each treatment.

Reiki is optimally offered in a complete treatment format but can also be applied to a particular part or parts of the body in brief treatments. Even moments of Reiki touch can be soothing in urgent situations.

What Happen in a Reiki Session?

Reiki is best held in a peaceful environment, but can be done anywhere. The patient sits in a comfortable chair or lies fully dressed on a bed. Music may or may not be there, depending on the preference of the patient.

For 2 to 5 minutes, the practitioner places the hand lightly on or across certain parts of the head, limbs and torso with different hand forms. The hands can be placed around 20 different parts of the body.

If a serious injury occurs, such as a burn, the hands can be held over the wound.

While the practitioner holds his hands lightly on or over his body, energy is transferred. The practitioner's hands can be moist and tingling during this process.

The practitioner holds each hand position until he feels that the power has stopped flowing.

When the practitioner thinks warmth or energy has fallen in his hands, he will withdraw his hand and put it on another part of the body.

Some Techniques in Reiki

The techniques include the following:

- Centering
- Clearing
- Extracting harmful energies
- Beaming
- Infusing
- Ranking and smoothing the aura

Some Reiki practitioner will use crystals and chakra healing walls since they find these can heal or protect a house against negative energy.

Nevertheless, Annie Harrington, President of the Reiki Federation of the United

Kingdom, said: "We do not use crystals, wands or powders as a general rule. One of the advantages of Reiki healing is remote healing (where Reiki is sent over several miles), so that many practitioners are helping out with the use of crystals. The number of sessions depends on what a customer wants to do. Many clients prefer a single meeting, while others want to focus on a certain topic with a series of sessions.

Reiki sessions can last for 20-80 minutes. The number of sessions vary and it is dependent on what the customer wishes to achieve. Some customers prefer to go for a session while other go for series of sessions to achieve their goals.

Becoming a Reiki Practitioner

To become a Reiki practitioner, no preparation, training or experience is required in order to enter into the Reiki practice or "attunement process." The masters are said to transfer the "attunement" energy and healing techniques to the student during this process, considered to be a "powerful spiritual experience."

Training in Reiki varies, but most students learn about the following:

Energy all around the body

How to work with healing energy

The ethics of working with customers

Preparing for attunement process includes fasting for two to three days, reflecting on Nature, meditation, and emotional reaction.

There are three mastery levels. Those who attain the "Master" level can educate others and can heal like a form of prayer from far away.

Benefits of Reiki

Reiki can help enhance the immune system, release the body toxins, stimulate good circulation and digestion, soothe mind and emotions and restore harmony and balance.

- Reiki is extremely beneficial for pregnant women during pregnancy. It can ease tension; it can relax the mother and help the unborn child greatly. It can also help waiting mothers with anxiety, fatigue, sorrow and pain.

- Reiki can be very relaxing and can help to recover post-natal and even post-natal.

- Reiki is gentle and calming with babies and children. In general, babies and children love Reiki and often respond to it very quickly. Treatments are usually shorter than for an adult.

- Reiki can work well with stress-related conditions like migraines, insomnia, anxiety and high blood pressure for stress, tension, and fatigue. It can reduce muscle tension, tiredness and pain, and boost energy levels.

- Reiki encourages natural healing processes of the body for injuries, procedures and trauma, helping speed up recovery from an incident, procedure or injury.

- Acute pain can be quickly relieved by Reiki for pain. Chronic, more profound conditions can also react well, but additional treatments are needed to get to the root of the problem.

- Mental / emotional imbalances can be used to respond to reiki as well as compulsive and suppressive behavioral patterns through emotional problems such as frustration, grief, anxiety, depression, and fear. This can make Reiki very helpful in cases of dependency on drugs or alcohol or nutritional disorders.

- At the end of ones life, sometimes in case of terminal illness, the development of the disease cannot be reversed. However, in these cases Reiki can help to improve the quality of the time left and bring peace and acceptance to the end of the life of a person.

Chapter 2: Chi, Chakras, And Reiki

Chi is synonymous with breath in the Chinese language. The idea of chi exists in many other cultures and goes by other names. In India, chi is called prana; in Hawaii, it is called mana; in Japan it is ki. Chi is the invisible electromagnetic life force within all living beings. In living creatures, energy flows through not only from physical nourishment but pathways in the body called meridians and energy centers called chakras.

Chi is not created or destroyed; instead, it transforms endlessly and changes its manifestation. Chi may also be spelled ch'i, qi, or ki, but they all mean the same thing. Our internal organs—heart, liver, kidney, and glands—refine this energy and send its power to the higher functions of our brain, thus creating our cognitive thoughts, conscious and subconscious dreams, and emotions. From this emerges the human will to live or die, the power to love, live, and breathe in harmony with the universe. In terms of the human body, strong chi denotes a being who is alive, alert, and present in the moment. A weak chi, conversely, can lead to fatigue and illness.

Chi goes beyond the physical, however, to the mental and the spiritual, because human functions go beyond just the physical aspect of being. Unbalanced mental chi can bring feelings of distress or frustration while developing mental chi can bring clarity, balance, and focus to your life. Spiritual chi brings about higher states of consciousness and feelings of higher purpose and spiritual well-being. It is important to understand the power of chi, as it is the energy force that is worked in Reiki and energy healing arts.

The Chakras

As previously mentioned, the chakras are important as they are energy pathways in the body. The word chakra is a Sanskrit word meaning wheel, circle, or disc, as the circle is the perceived shape of chakras, and are often depicted as circles in drawings. A chakra is a subtle energy center of the body and a part of the larger energy center called the energosoma. The chakra system is like a spiritual nervous system that connects to all parts of the body. Many cultures, philosophies, religions, and alternative medicines believe that chakras are connected to overall health and well-being.

There are seven main chakras that are more commonly known and used in practice, but in reality, there are thousands of secondary and peripheral chakras. Each chakra aligns with a part of the body and is represented by a color. Imagine the spine as a stem. The chakras, therefore, would be the flowers growing out of the stem, through the body, and out into the aura (the energy field that surrounds the body). The main seven chakras and their corresponding chakras are (from the head working downwards):

Coronochakra: the crown chakra (Sahasrara). The only chakra to be found outside of the physical body, this is located just above the crown of the head. This chakra is associated with higher consciousness, pure unconditional love and a state of quintessential being. There are no physical organs it is associated with, but it is connected to reenergizing the brain, and the color is usually depicted as light purple, indigo, or white. A blockage in this chakra can lead to headaches, insomnia, anxiety, and depression.

Frontochakra: the third eye chakra (Ajna). The third eye chakra is located in the center of the brain, at the crossroads between the eyes and just above the ears. This chakra represents intelligence and wisdom, imagination, and an ability to analyze and perceive truth in the world. The color is a deep purple and is associated with the pituitary gland, the nose, ears, and the pineal gland, a small, pea-shaped gland in the brain. Issues with the third eye chakra may cause headaches, insomnia, anxiety, and depression, the same issues related to crown chakra blockages.

Laryngochakra: the throat chakra (Vishudha). Located at the throat, this chakra represents communication, creativity, truth, and dependability. The color blue is usually associated with the throat chakra and the associated organs are the thyroid, hypothalamus, throat, and mouth. Throat chakra blockages cause issues with communication, addictive behaviors that keep you from speaking your truth, respiratory diseases, dental issues, low self-esteem, hostility, and resentment.

Cardiochakra: the heart chakra (Anahata). The heart chakra, not surprisingly, is located near the heart. This chakra represents love, unconditional love, acceptance, empathy, and presentiment.

Green is the color of the heart chakra (not red, as is the color usually associated with the heart) and the organs it governs are the heart, the arms, hands, and the circulatory system. When the heart chakra is out of alignment, it can lead you to feel depressed, fearful, resentful, and may lead to heart disease and other cardiac disorders.

Splenochakra: the solar plexus chakra (Manipura). This chakra is located by (not in) the belly button. The solar plexus chakra represents our willpower and ability to stand up for ourselves. The color is yellow and associated with the pancreas, liver, spleen, and stomach. If the solar plexus chakra is unbalanced, it may lead to feelings of insecurity, controlling behaviors, and digestive disorders.

Umbilicochakra: sacral (Svadisthana). This chakra is also called the sacral chakra, as it is located near the sacrum, a large piece of bone at the base of the spine, and above the coccyx, or tailbone. This chakra represents desire and pleasure, spiritual and emotional balance, and sexuality. This chakra is usually depicted with the color orange and the reproductive organs, bladder, and prostate. An imbalance of the sacral chakra can lead to abuse of food, sex, or alcohol; sexual or reproductive disorders; uncertainty; envy; and low self-esteem.

Sexochakra: the root chakra (Muladhara). The root chakra is located at the base or root of the body, called the perineum. This chakra represents grounding, and basic survival instincts, like food and shelter. It also affects our passion, imagination and creativity, youthfulness, and vitality. The root chakra is represented by the color red and is associated with the spinal column, adrenal glands, kidneys, colon, and legs. This chakra centers on physical strength, sexuality, and the fight or flight response that is stimulated when we sense danger. An imbalance of the root chakra leads to fear, victimization, selfishness, violence, and lower back, feet, and leg pain.

How the chakras work with Reiki

As stated previously, Reiki works to free energy blockages in the body. A blockage is when the energy in the body gets constricted. These blockages are associated with the chakras, and Reiki, therefore, helps clear these blockages to balance your energy, and in turn, your chakras.

Chakras do not work independently of each other; instead, they all work together as a part of a larger energy system. If one chakra is imbalanced, all of your chakras will be out of alignment. While chakras do all work together, each chakra has a role in the balance of the energy in your mind, body, and spirit.

Because of the stress of daily life, it is not uncommon for one or more of our chakras to fall out of alignment. This imbalance shows up as physical or mental symptoms that correspond to a specific chakra. Reiki practitioners believe that physical symptoms that show up without injury are due to emotional blockages deep within.

A Reiki practitioner can find your imbalances and help clear them with one or more Reiki sessions designed around your specific issues. Reiki helps clear the blockages in your chakras to allow for a more peaceful existence without the physical and mental anguish that comes with blockages.

Chapter 3: Reiki And The Science Behind It

Research and Findings to Support the Science of Reiki's Benefits

In recent decades, Reiki has grown in popularity as a form of therapy and treatment that helps many people with a wide range of health and medical conditions.

While it is considered an alternative therapy, it has been used with positive results that complement and improve the effectiveness of conventional Western medicine.

There are some studies that indicate a positive effect on cancer patients who receive Reiki treatments, including pain relief, reduced anxiety and less stress overall.

Reduced pain and tension, in general, are also benefits that have been reported by people who have experienced the powerful therapeutic effects of Reiki.

In the United States, Reiki has grown significantly in the 1990s, evolving from a historical discovery and concept to a new, modern way to heal with universal energy.

Due to the positive feedback from people using and practicing Reiki, it has increased in popularity and now widely offered in hospitals across the U.S. and in other countries as well.

Reiki provides a gentle, relaxing therapy that gives relief during difficult experiences patients may undergo in hospitals and clinics, such as cancer treatment (radiation, chemotherapy), surgery as well as other procedures (CAT scans, MRIs) and medications.

There are other benefits that support the use and practice of Reiki, either in a hospital, clinical setting, or a less formal space:

- Reiki is completely risk-free and does not cause any harm nor side effects to the person receiving treatment. In other words, even people who may be skeptical at first will give it a try, because there is nothing to risk or lose.

Most, if not all people, have a pleasant experience during their first treatment.

- There is always a benefit from Reiki, whether it's relaxation and stress reduction or a reduction in pain.

Some people have reported the remission of disease or reduction of certain ailments, as a result of Reiki, though results can vary from one individual to the next.

- Reiki is not used to substitute conventional therapy, but rather, as a support for the body's natural ability to heal and improve your health overall.

This is another reason why it is strongly supported by the medical community and hospital network in the U.S., as it can alleviate the stress and negative symptoms often associated with some treatments.

It gives patients something to enjoy and look forward to, after a difficult day of treatment.

- Some people report feeling more energetic and less fatigued after a session of Reiki. Chronic fatigue is a condition that affects a significant number of people, and many will take prescription medication or other forms of therapy to cope.

Reiki can also provide additional support and energy while delivering this healing effect with a calm, peacefulness, opening, and increasing the flow of energy without added tension.

- Reiki can be used on everyone of all ages, backgrounds, and abilities.

Since there is no risk of harm or side effects at all, anyone from a newborn baby, someone who is pregnant, to someone of advanced age can benefit from Reiki.

Pets are also great candidates for treatment, as well.

Reiki is also beneficial for people who may not have a specific condition or medical issue but would like to experience a general sense of relaxation and peace.

Most people experience stress on a regular basis, and this often becomes chronic, even when we are unaware of it.

We may hold onto tension and worry too often, or find it difficult to unwind and relax, even when there is an opportunity to do so.

Reading and learning about Reiki is a good start, and speaking with friends, colleagues or acquaintances who may have experienced a Reiki therapy session, or took a class themselves, will give you a better idea of what to expect before you begin.

Chapter 4: An Overview Of Reiki.

REIKI'S ORIGIN:

Reiki was discovered in Japan in the mid-19th century and was brought to the United States in the early 1940's. From a single practitioner in the United States, the Reiki phenomenon has grown to over a million practitioners world-wide. I am one of them.

I was first introduced to Reiki in 1996 and am now a certified Reiki Master-Teacher as well as a certified Animal Reiki Practitioner. This means that I am qualified to conduct trainings, attunements (initiations – more on these later), and treatments for both people and animals.

I have been owned by cats for more than 20 years. Phantom, my handsome Russian Blue, is sitting next to me as I work on this book, freely mowing his advice. Phantom is a lap-lover and the happy recipient of many Reiki treatments. Unlike his human who is prone to exhibiting a "Reiki snore" when getting a treatment, Phantom simply closes his eyes and "zones out" in bliss.

REIKI AS AN ENERGY:

The word "Reiki" comes from several Japanese Kanji symbols, which translate to "universal life energy". This is the energy, which animates all life forms.

Many forces cause disharmony within animated energy systems: mental and emotional disturbances, physical trauma, and environmental influences to name a few. These disharmonies can eventually be manifested within the body (both animal and human) as diseases or undesired behaviors. Reiki helps to minimize or eliminate the underlying disharmonies.

REIKI AS A SYSTEM OF HEALING:

Reiki energy automatically switches "on" whenever a practitioner's hands are placed on or near any intended recipient. No conscious effort or intent is required. During a treatment, both the practitioner and the recipient may feel sensations of warmth, cold, or tingling (or they may feel nothing at all). The absence of such sensations does not mean that the Reiki energy is not working: Reiki is ALWAYS flowing.

Reiki is not a spiritual belief system; it does not have to be believed or understood for it to work effectively. The only requirement is that the recipient must accept the healing energy. The Reiki Healing System does offer five principles of living that are easily stated, but are more difficult to live up to on a daily basis.

The Reiki Principles are re-stated here as affirmations (positive statements made in the present tense as if they are already complete) along with a trigger word for each one that is used during meditations:

Just for today, I am free of anger (LOVE).

- Just for today, I am free of worry (SERENITY).

- Just for today, I am kind to all living things (COMPASSION).

- Just for today, I do my work honestly (INTEGRITY).

- Just for today, I am grateful for my many blessings (GRATITUDE).

Reiki is also a self-directed energy; you do not need to know where to direct the energy. There are no harmful side effects from Reiki, but there can be some short-term discomfort as the body begins to heal.

Reiki energy is not a naturally occurring state for humans. Acquiring the ability to channel energy to others requires training and an attunement (initiation) conducted by a certified Reiki Master-Teacher. Once attuned, you will have the ability to channel Reiki energy for the rest of your life. There are three levels of Reiki attunements:

- Reiki I attunes you to the energy and teaches you how to provide hands-on treatments.

- Reiki II teaches you three sacred Reiki symbols that: increase Reiki's strength, focus on mental-emotional healing, and allow the sending of Reiki energy across time and space.

- Reiki II is the Master-Teacher level where you learn how to transmit attunements and how to train others.

Chapter 5: The 21-Day Cleansing Process

Or Reiki

Reiki can affect every area of your life. Reiki works by increasing the vibrations of energy within your body, bringing you closer to your natural self. Many practitioners of Reiki also state that they are able to manifest their desires and goals into reality with the focus that they derive from its practice. Any imbalance between you and your universe can be restored easily with regular practice of Reiki. Some even believe that you can balance the events of your past and present life with Reiki, too.

But, on the flip side, many people feel like their life has become much harder after Reiki attunement. This is because of the sensitivity that you develop towards smaller issues around you. You see, Reiki depends upon the emotional blocks that are seated deep inside you. When these blocks open up, you become more and more sensitive to any additional problem or issue within your body or even around you.

This can cause a lot of stress that begins to accumulate inside your body. And, when you do not address this stress in time, it can even begin to affect your organs after a certain point. That is when we start to fall ill. You see, stress in any form is toxic for your body. You need to clear the stress out to purify your emotional blocks as well as your body.

When you initiate the Reiki cleansing process, you will feel a lot of flu -like symptoms. It feels like your lymphatic system is swollen, your joints begin to ache and your mind just closes itself. Most often, when people experience this, the first thing that they do is take several medicines and get into bed. Now, this is not the solution when your issue is related to your Reiki energy. What will happen is a relapse of the condition. This is because the toxins are unable to leave the body. When you are sleeping all day, you will neither perspire, nor will you pass urine. The moment you resume activity, you feel like you are recovering simply because your bodily functions are restored. Now, you can even cleanse your body and your mind through a 21-day cleansing process.

Purifying the physical self

When you are using Reiki to cleanse the body, flu like symptoms are common. You may experience fever, muscle pain, headaches, cough, diarrhea and several other symptoms. As these toxins are being removed from your body, you will also notice a great difference in your metabolism. As the Reiki energy cleanses your chakras, you will feel them vibrating and sensations of spinning are experienced in these areas.

To make sure that the effect of this energy is reduced you can perform self Reiki in areas that show maximum symptoms. You can even try a few mild exercises, take long walks, get some fresh air and drink lots of fresh water. Fruits and vegetables and juices are great for your body too.

Purifying your emotional self

When you emotionally cleanse yourself, you will see that several deeply seated emotions will emerge. You may feel a magnified sense of frustration, anger, grief etc. These are the emotions that you have kept suppressed for a really long time. They could also be from very significant incidents in your life. The important thing to do is to disconnect your present self from these emotions. Do not allow yourself to connect these emotions to your current personal situations and life. Placing blame on other people, etc. should not be practiced when you are feeling this surge of emotions.

In order to feel some relief from these intense emotions, just place one hand on your forehead and one hand on your navel. While you do this, focus on your crown chakra. Imagine a white light circulating throughout your body and when you feel it exiting your body, let it out with a loud "Bah" noise. Keep doing this till you feel at peace. You can also take long baths with bath salts or Epsom salts. This will get all your intense emotions out and will cleanse you from within.

Purifying your mind

When you purify your mind with the energy of Reiki, you will notice that certain habits and behaviors will surface. You will get some addictive desires to beverages, nicotine, caffeine, food and other things that you could have been addicted to in the past. This is actually a way for the whole habit to be removed from all the levels of your being. It is not necessary to be hard on yourself. Take note of them and just let them go slowly.

Practice all the Reiki positions directed at the head. Make sure that you are kind to yourself. Pamper yourself during this phase and keep giving yourself a lot of positive messages and affirmations.

Spiritual purification

This is the last stage of the purification process. You will see yourself challenging your own beliefs about religion, relationships and life in general. In fact, this is when you actually begin to prioritize your life. It will become clearer to you about what is really important in your life and what makes you happy. These are new building blocks of your personality and will remain with you forever.

When you reach the last stage of cleansing, make sure that you spend a lot of time performing head positions with your palm.

During this cleansing process, it is the Reiki energy that is working vigorously to make you the best version of yourself in terms of your physical, emotional, spiritual and mental aspects of life. So, basically, you are able to get a whole different perspective on your own life. With all the negative thoughts and sensations gone, you become more sensitive and are able to impart your Reiki energy a lot more effectively. It also makes each practice more meaningful and fruitful as you only imbibe the strong positive vibrations of Reiki.

Chapter 6: Chakras And Auras

There are seven main chakras of the human body, but before we get into that, let us first explore what a chakra is. Chakra is a word derived from the Sanskrit language that translates to wheel. Each chakra is its own wheel within the human body that is propelled by energy. Depending upon the balance within your body, your chakras may move faster or slower. When one wheel is out of balance, the rest of the wheels are affected.

Every chakra within our body has a corresponding physical component. Those seven components are our sensory, breathing, circulation, digestion, reproduction, and secretion systems; as well as the seventh chakra located within the brain.

The chakras of the physical body are:

The Root Chakra – Located within the large intestines and the rectum. Influences the function of the kidneys.

The Naval Chakra – Corresponds to the reproductive system (testicles and ovaries) and the bladder and kidneys.

The Solar Plexus Chakra – Related to the gall bladder, liver, stomach, spleen, and the small intestines.

The Heart Chakra–Corresponds to the heart and arms.

The Throat Chakra – Relates to the lungs and throat.

The Third Eye (Forehead) – Corresponds to your brain; your nose; your eyes; your face; and so on.

The Crown Chakra – This is not related to any part of the body but encompasses the entire body.

In Reiki, chakras are focused upon within the person being healed, in order to bring balance back to the chakra affected, so that the rest of the chakras can fall back in line.

Auras relate to chakras in the sense that each chakra controls a different type of aura. There are seven auras within the human body known as auric bodies. The aura is the electromagnetic field surrounding the body. There is something known as an auric egg, which is around two to three feet in diameter, and it emits from the body and extends above the head and into the ground.

The seven auric layers interrelate to one another, and if there is an imbalance in one layer, it affects the others. Those seven layers, all different, pertain to a person's emotions, thinking behavior, health, and feelings. The seven different auric bodies are as follows:

Physical Auric Body – Pleasure, health, the physical comforts.

Etheric Auric Body – Self-love, response and also acceptance.

Vital Auric Body – The rational mind pertaining to situations. Defining a situation in a clear, rational, linear way.

Astral Auric Body – The emotional body with relation to others such as loving friends and family.

Lower Mental Auric Body – The divine will within that makes commitments to speak the truth and follow it.

Higher Mental Auric Body – Spiritual ecstasy and divine love.

Spiritual Auric Body – Serenity, the divine mind. To be able to connect with and understand the great universal pattern.

Each of these auras can have a different color. When we are able to see these colors, we can determine what a person is feeling in that moment and get a deeper sense of their soul. A process known as Kirlian photography is able to capture the colors of the aura around the human body, as well as around animals; plants; as well as objects.

Here is a list of varying colors and also what each of them represents within the aura.

Red – Related to the physical body such as the heart and circulation.

Deep Red – A person with this aura color is strong-willed and with great survival abilities; realistic; active; and in totality, a grounded person.

Muddied Red – People with this aura are angry and repelling.

Clear Red – People with this type of aura have passion; lots of energy; and feel powerful.

Pink and Bright – Indicative of a clairaudience, pink is a sign of someone who is tender, loving, sensitive, artistic, pure, affectionate, and compassionate.

Dark or Murky Pink – Dishonest and immature.

Orange Red – A person who is confident and creative.

Orange – The orange aura is related to the reproductive system and emotions. It is a color of vigor, good health, vitality, and excitement.

Orange/Yellow – Someone who is creative; detail-oriented; intelligent; having a scientific mind; and also a perfectionist.

Yellow – This aura color relates to the life energy and the spleen. It is indicative of inspiration; creativity; optimism; as well as intelligence.

Light or Pale – Someone with this aura is experiencing a positive excitement about new ideas and spiritual awareness. They are hopeful and full of optimism.

Bright – Someone with aura fears losing control and respect within a personal or business relationship.

Golden – Someone who has been inspired.

Dark/Brown – Someone who is feeling stressed out about learning so many things all at the same time; actually struggling to fit all the things in at once.

Green – This aura relates to the heart and lungs, and indicates someone who is healthy, comfortable, and has a lot of love for people; animals; as well as nature.

Emerald – This person is a healer and centers their life around love.

Yellow-Green – A communicative person who is creative when it comes to matters of the heart.

Dark – Someone who is feeling jealous or resentful; blaming other people for their personal problems; and feeling very insecure. Such persons suffer low self-esteem and lack understanding of personal responsibility.

Turquoise – People with this aura are actually sensitive; great healers; therapists; and also compassionate. The turquoise color relates to the immune system.

Blue – This color relates to the throat as well as the thyroid. It points to a person who is calm; collected; and also caring.

Soft – This is indicative of peacefulness as well as clarity. A person who possesses this aura has honesty and is great in communication.

Royal – This person is a clairvoyant and highly spiritual in nature. They're generous and on the right path.

Dark – People with this aura have a fear of the future and a fear of expressing themselves.

Indigo – This color relates to the third eye and the pituitary gland.

Violet – Related to the crown and pineal gland, this color indicates someone who is idealistic and in tune with their self.

Lavender – Someone with this color is a visionary and also a daydreamer; one with vivid imagination.

Silver – People with this color are having an awakening of the cosmic mind.

Bright – People with this color are receptive and bright.

Dark – If gray clusters are seen within specific parts of your body, it is an indication of a health related problem emerging. People with such indicators have residual fear.

Gold – A golden aura means that this person is experiencing enlightenment and they're being guided by a higher power.

Black – This is usually indicative of an arising health problem and long-term inability to forgive others. People with this aura usually experience past life events that are unsavory.

White – Someone who is pure in nature. If there are sparkles, there might be a higher being nearby or the person may become pregnant soon.

Earth Colors – They're a good sign and they represent love of nature.

Rainbow – Someone who is a Reiki healer or one you can call a star person; a person in their 1st reincarnation on earth.

Pastel – A person who needs serenity and is sensitive.

Dirty Brown – Someone who is insecure.

Dirty Gray – A person who is guarded.

Now that you're comfortable with what and where the seven chakras are located as well as their corresponding auras, let's move on to symbols in the Reiki practice.

Chapter 7: History Of Reiki

The Reiki strategy for heling was established on the disclosure and comprehension of the body's vitality framework. Reiki Practitioners endeavor to improve wellbeing and personal satisfaction by offering Reiki vitality and reestablishing harmony. Reiki is utilized in self-care, for consideration of one's family and is offered in private practice, in emergency clinics and restorative environments as an aide and steady treatment to health and conventional medicinal consideration. The type of Reiki that numerous individuals practice today, Usui Reiki, has been used for more than one hundred years.

The Founder of Reiki

The historical backdrop of Usui Reiki starts with its founder, Dr. Mikao Usui. Now and then called the Usui Sensei, Dr. Mikao Usui was born in a well-off Buddhist family in

1865. Dr. Usui's family had the option to give their child balanced instruction for that time. As a tyke, Dr. Usui grew up in a Buddhist religious community where he was shown hand to hand fighting, swordsmanship, and the Japanese type of Chi Kung, known as Kiko.

All through his training, Dr. Usui had an enthusiasm for medicine, brain research and religious philosophy. It was this intrigue that incited him to look for an approach to heal himself as well as other people utilizing the laying on of hands. It was his longing to discover a curing technique that was unattached to a particular religion and religious conviction, so his framework would be available to everybody.

Dr. Usui voyaged a lot during his lifetime. He concentrated mending frameworks of various types and held various callings including journalist, secretary, teacher, community worker and watchman. At long last, he turned into a Buddhist cleric/priest and lived in a religious community.

Otherworldly Awakening and Development of Reiki

At some point during his long stretches of preparing in the religious community, Dr. Usui went to his very own preparation rediscovery course in a cavern on Mount Kurama. For 21 days, Dr. Usui fasted, contemplated and prayed. Moreover, on the morning of the twenty-first day, Dr. Usui encountered an occasion that would change his life for eternity. He saw old Sanskrit images that helped him build up the arrangement of healing he had been attempting to design. Usui Reiki was conceived.

After his otherworldly awakening on Mount Kurama, Dr. Usui built up a facility for curing and educating in Kyoto. As the act of Usui Reiki was spreading, Dr. Usui ended up being known for his healing practice.

Other commendable Development about Reiki

Hands on mending has been logically demonstrated to be viable in speeding up healing.

A Reiki treatment bolsters the entire individual including body, feelings, brain and soul making numerous helpful impacts.

On a physical level Reiki enables reduction of pain, quickens the mending time of bones and wounds, loosens up muscles and decreases the tissue formation on wounds. It is conceivable to ameliorate the negative symptoms of medication, for example, chemotherapy and radiation. Colds, flus, honeybee stings, coronary illness - numerous physical conditions - can be treated with Reiki.

On a psychological and passionate level uneasiness is diminished, feelings of prosperity expanded and another degree of unwinding can be felt. At this level of profound unwinding a rebalancing of energies happens and the common mending capacity of the body is improved.

On a spiritual level, patients have expressed that they feel reawakened and restored after a full-body session.

How is a Reiki treatment given?

A run of the mill Reiki treatment will see the customer lying fully dressed on a back-rub table. It is additionally possible to give a Reiki treatment to a customer sitting or standing. The professional places his or her hands on, or close to the customer's body in a progression of hand positions from the head to the feet holding them for 2 to 10 mins, depending upon how much time is required at each hand arrangement. The treatment will commonly last somewhere in the range of 45 mins to an hour and may incorporate input acquired by the expert during the treatment. A customer may refer to their professional for a fortnightly appointment, for some time or may find one session enough for all the vital advantages. Reiki experts are able to give separation mending, meaning you could be anyplace on the planet and get healing from your expert.

What does a Reiki treatment feel like?

Everybody will have a somewhat extraordinary encounter. Anyway, regularly, individuals experience a stronger feeling of unwinding. I, personally, feel a stunning sparkling brilliance or vitality traveling through my body, here and there in floods and it will move through me and surround me. Others will have dreams or feel like they are drifting over their body. Where the specialist feels blockages in a subject's vitality (and will invest time clearing that blockage), the patient may feel an underlying largeness followed by a discharge and stream of vitality. It isn't unusual for customers to encounter a passionate discharge, as enthusiastic disturbance is brought to the surface and discharged.

Reiki is likewise a profound practice that develops genuine feelings of serenity, improves our wellbeing and essentialness and encourages mental prosperity. Every day self-Reiki medication is an attraction of health: the foundation of thinking about ourselves and attracting consistency and wellbeing on all levels. Reiki is the gift that keeps on giving.

The word "Reiki" implies soul vitality or the vitality of the Universe, which is found in every single living thing, plants and creatures notwithstanding. As individuals, we are altogether brought into the world with Reiki; an attunement or reiju is everything necessary to enable us to actuate or stir this capacity and recall all that we are able to do.

The training started with Mikao Usui in Japan back in the mid-1920s. Usui's involvement of illumination and deep-rooted profound practice drove him to build up the healing technique we currently know as Reiki. He created Reiki as a profound practice to develop significant serenity in this way expanding wellbeing and prosperity. Usui Sensei skilled us with the Reiki statutes as devices for mental prosperity and profound development.

The Reiki strategy for healing was based on the disclosure and comprehension of the body's vitality framework. Reiki Practitioners endeavor to improve wellbeing and personal satisfaction by offering Reiki vitality and reestablishing harmony. Reiki is utilized in self-care, for consideration of one's family and is offered in private practice and in emergency clinics as an assistant and steady treatment to wellbeing and customary medicinal consideration. The type of Reiki that numerous individuals practice today, Usui Reiki, has been used for more than one hundred years.

As we stated, the historical backdrop of Usui Reiki starts with its originator, Dr. Mikao Usui.

In the mid-1990s there were discoveries of Usui's unique Reiki lessons. The commemoration of Usui was found by western instructors and many people from Reiki's missing connections were revealed. Disclosures incorporated the revelation of a living Reiki practice in Japan, with extra strategies as instructed by the Reiki Gakkai (Reiki Learning Society). Some of Usui's notes and manuals were likewise shared and this prompted more noteworthy discoveries which were later made and became largely accessible. Western Reiki instructors increased new data seeing the framework as it had been taught in Japan and this was sorted out with set up frameworks of Reiki in the West.

Usui's Students

On September 1_{st} 1923, the devasting Kanto earthquake struck Tokyo and the surrounding regions. A large portion of the center piece of Tokyo was leveled and completely pulverized by flame. More than 140,000 individuals were murdered. In one case, 40,000 individuals were burned when a flame tornado cleared over the open territory where they had looked for shelter. Tragically the quake struck in the late morning, exactly when peoples' charcoal flame broils were set to prepare lunch. 3,000,000 homes were shattered, leaving endless amounts of people broke. More than 50,000 individuals endured serious wounds. The open water and sewage frameworks were destroyed and it took a very long time for re-working to happen.

Considering this disaster, Usui and his students offered Reiki to numerous unfortunate casess. His facility turned out to be too little to even consider handling the crowds of patients, so in February 1924, he manufactured another center in Nakano, outside Tokyo. His notoriety spread rapidly all through Japan and he started accepting solicitations from everywhere throughout the nation to come and show his healing techniques. Usui was granted a Kun San from the Emperor, which is a high grant (much like a privileged doctorate), given to the individuals who had done respectable work. His acclaim before long spread all through the district. Numerous noticeable healers and doctors started mentioning lessons from him.

Usui rapidly turned out to be head over heels as solicitations for instructing Reiki kept on arriving. He travelled predominantely all through Japan which was not a simple endeavor back then, to instruct and give Reiki attunements. This began to negatively affect his wellbeing and he started encountering light strokes from pressure. On March 9_{th}, 1926, while in Fukuyama, Usui unfortunately died of a lethal stroke. He was 62 years old.

It is said that Usui instructed Reiki to a little more than 2000 individuals and out of these successors a few sources state he prepared 22 to educator level(Shinpiden). Huge numbers of these students started their very own centers and established Reiki schools and social orders.

By the 1940s there were around 40 Reiki schools spread all over Japan. The vast majority of these schools taught the strategy for Reiki that Usui had created.

Dr Chujiro Hayashi

The ancestry of most of Western Reiki experts springs from Chuijro Hayashi. Hayashi taught with Mikao Usui for around ten months preceding Usui's passing. He is known to have changed a portion of the strategies of Usui.

Chuijro Hayashi was born in 1879. At some point, in 1925 Chuijro Hayashi met Usui. Chuijro had ascended to be an authority in the Imperial Navy and had prepared in Western and Chinese Medicine. In June of

1925, Hayashi got his instructor's preparation in Usui's framework. A few sources state that Chuijro Hayashi was a Methodist Christian, a reality affirmed one of his Shoden/Okudent understudies, Mrs.Yamaguchi. Different sources state that he was a Soto Zen specialist who used the acts of Shinto. For all we know, he may have been both as this would be flawlessly as per Japanese ways to deal with religion. As a Christian, Hayashi would have taken in the rearranged type of Reiki.

Before his demise on tenth May 1940 Hayashi coached 13 students to the educator level, inccluding Hawayo Takata in 1938.

Mrs. Takata - Usui Shiki Ryoh

Hawayo Kawamura (her original last name) was brought into the world on December 25th 1900 in Hanamaula, Kauai, Hawaii. On the tenth of March 1917 she married her significant other, Saichi Takata. They had two little girls, one named Alice Takata-Furumoto, who later had a little girl named Phyllis Furumoto.

It is because of Mrs. Takata that Reiki is outstanding and wide spread all through the world. Mrs. Takata officially brought Reiki to America at the beginning of the 1970s and during a multiyear time frame, brought 22 Western students to the instructor level. Her style of Reiki was created from the learnings she recieved from Dr Hayashi.

It was following the death of her significant other in 1930 and her sister's in 1935 that Hawayo Takata chose to go to Japan to visit her folks. Because of the work she put into help her family and the sadness caused by her loses, Takata's wellbeing had started to suffer. She has booked an appointment in Japan to check her medical issues. Just before the appointmen she heard the voice of her dead spouse, saying that the practice she's chosen was a bit much and that there was another way. This determined her to talk with her primary care physician about elective medicine, so he suggested her Hayashi's Reiki Clinic. Hawayo Takata gotten day by day medications at stayed at this facility for a period of four months and during this time her symptoms totally subsided.

This drove Hawayo Takata to take Reiki One preparing (Shoden) with Hayashi on December 10th, 1935. She examined the principal level with him for barely one year. In 1937, Mrs. Takata got the subsequent level, Okuden. Soon after this, she came back to Hawaii. Half a month later, Hayashi visited Mrs. Takata with his little girl and remained until February 1938. During this time Hayashi made Mrs. Takata a Reiki educator.

Somewhere in the range of 1940 and 1970, Mrs. Takata ran a few Reiki centers and showed numerous classes in Hawaii. In 1973 she showed her five stars in the United States. In December of 1980 Mrs. Takata has passed. Much appreciation and affirmation are perceived for Mrs. Takata in empowering Reiki to spread all through the world. Without her, the arrangement of Reiki may have right up 'til the present stayed obscure but to a chosen few in Japan.

Dr Usui's Original Reiki Teachings

The most profound otherworldly practices and procedures of the Japanese conventions have stayed behind Japan's shut Reiki society. The first Reiki of Mikao Usui still thrives in Japan yet is impressively unique practically speaking. Outside of Japan there are just three authorized educators of the pre-1922 framework – one of whom is an individual from The Reiki Guild.

Chapter 8: Medical Concerns

In most situations Reiki is indicated, meaning it is appropriate to use for the reasons the person is seeking treatment. There are however some things to take into consideration prior to a Reiki session. Below is a list of medical conditions that require caution and special attention. As a practitioner it is up to you to follow your training and intuition when deciding if Reiki is appropriate or not.

Pace maker- Clients with a pacemaker may receive a Reiki treatment with the area around the Heart Chakra being avoided. The reason for this is because the energy frequency that flows from a practitioners hands may be enough to cause palpitations and "hiccups" in the pacemaker function. As a result it is best to not perform Reiki in the area above or around the pacemaker as a precautionary measure.

Heart Palpitations- As mentioned above with the use of pacemakers, Reiki has been known to sometimes increase heart palpitations in those that are prone to this condition. While it does not happen every time, there is no way to know if it is the Reiki producing this effect, or something else. Some people with palpitations have reported a decrease in episodes. As a precaution, keep a clear line of communication open with the client and encourage them to tell you immediately if they begin to have any palpitations.

Anxiety- Levels of anxiety vary. When working on clients with anxiety be sure to ask what they would like for you to do in case of an anxiety or panic attack during treatment. Because Reiki is changing the vibrational energy of the client, it can stir-up feelings of anxiety. It is important to discuss this with your client prior to treatment.

PTSD- It is important to discuss what to do in case a client's PTSD is triggered during a session. As with anxiety, it can be stirred-up during treatment as the energy levels change within the body. It is also a common occurrence for the client and/or the practitioner to visualize the disturbing image that is haunting the client. Be aware during the treatment and know ahead of time what the client would like for you to do if they become distressed.

Mental Illness- In cases of severe mental illness such as schizophrenia or bipolar disorder use extreme caution. The difference in energy frequency can trigger an episode to flare, or cause them to become uncomfortable in the session. Talk with the client prior to treatment to develop a plan in case this should occur.

Remember the client has the right to refuse treatment or end a session at any time. In order to uphold professional standards, you should respect your client's wishes.

Chapter 9: Symbols

3.1. Description and meaning of energies carried by the symbols

So far I have never seen anyone either turning the Reiki symbols into sculptures or drawing them somewhere in public. I can only feel them as visualized light forms which carry the energy and the signature assigned to them. So, this is the part where we will talk about each symbol and their essential meanings so that you can use them in your everyday contact with the outer and inner world. The symbols are concentrated energy in a defined form and with a defined specific purpose. Dr. Usui never explained how these symbols were attained, but people who know them by the nature of things draw them without being taught how to do that. This is one of the clear evidence that the forms of symbols are based on the natural phenomenon of the visualization of light in a defined form. These symbols have been given to us and if we know how to awaken the symbols with their energy, we can become aware of them. Having studied various techniques of communicating with energies, I have found out that every person possesses their own symbol and that many of these symbols bear similarities. Often their form is spiral, that of lightening, light ball or light cloak, and all these forms are essential parts of the Reiki symbols. Due to being used for many years, the Reiki symbols have gained a high concentration of energy which makes them more efficient than our personal symbols. However, if you filled your personal symbol with energy every day, after some years of use it would contain substantial amount of energy needed to affect your surroundings successfully. We all know that each religion has its own symbols made in different sizes so that a religious person can connect themselves with that energy, thus devoting themselves to their religion.

The Reiki symbols help people to open themselves to the flow of energy, thus enabling them to become aware of their inner world with ease and to discover places where their being is welcome. A Reiki practitioner is a person who fits into time and place more smoothly and deals with life situations in a simpler way, without asking to be led all the time by other people. The symbols are here to clear the way for the flow of energy, so as to help the practitioner handle a certain situation. Obviously, the concentrated energy clears the way more effectively and this is why the symbols were created in the first place. Since we all add a part of ourselves and our life energy to the symbols with the constant communication with the outer energies of the Universe, the symbols possess an endless strength to affect what happens. The more time you spend with them, the more efficient they become in the task you assign them. Do not ever feel afraid of not knowing something, because if someone or something does not need Reiki symbols, the symbols will simply have no effects in that direction and they will return to you. These symbols do not impose themselves on other people. They just go there where they are needed, called for and accepted. You know that you cannot affect the people who do not want you or who are not related to you, regardless of the type of this relationship. The symbol will have effect on that part which is called 'the bond between you and that person', but it will not affect the other person if there is no relationship between the two of you. If you want to have effect on a person and you cannot do that for some reason, you will get a cold response on your palms and everything will be clear to you. There is no communication between you and that person.

You should just feel the information which has been sent to you; without any fear, everything is clear here! Spending time with the Reiki symbols you will learn to evaluate what it means when you are feeling 'cold', 'tepid' or 'warm'. Working with them will help you recognize new people coming into your life much faster. This works a bit differently with the people you have known for years, as there are long-standing habits in the behavioral patterns that you share, that is, there are the so-called routine hypocrisies that you are both used to. It is hard to change some habits, but if you use the symbols persistently, they will lead you to situations in which it will be possible to change even those old behavioral habits. Then you become the true Reiki practitioner. Bear in mind that the symbols will never let you down, especially if you spend time with them daily, since what happens between you and the symbols is love at first and all other sights, so just enjoy spending time with them!

3.2. First symbol: Cho–ku-rei

Represents: increase of energy, materialization; inviting cosmic energies to the physical level; it is used it to start and end Reiki treatments; it represents the capital letter at the beginning and the full stop at the end; it reinforces the existence on the material level, increases our inner strength and cures depression; first awakening; it opens the energy channel between us and a given location; and finally, after the exchange of energies, it breaks our connection to the place we have just explored.

At the beginning of your friendship with the first symbol, do not expect to be able to visualize it completely and to see its effect clearly. However, once you have spent time with Cho-ku-rei every day for 21 days, you will become aware of its effects and of how the outer world reacts to this symbol. This beauty of movement of the outer world at the moment when Cho-ku-rei appears keeps fascinating me again and again! The ease of removing the obstacles to react to certain situations or the clarity of movement to materialize what is touched by this symbol makes everyone feel confident that Reiki is very effective through the use and sending of the first symbol first, and then later of the other symbols. Obviously, you can send this symbol only to places within your sight, but this symbol is visibly active even within that distance. Send the first symbol playfully and with joy to all directions around you, and you will know that you are happy because Cho-ku-rei supports you and moves you on your journey along the rivers of life.

Cho bent sword, one that draws the bent line

ku breakthrough, so as to make something whole, in places where there is nothing rei outer energy, transcendental spirit, mysterious strength

It is always used as the switch bringing light to the world in which you make your way.

Cho-ku-rei

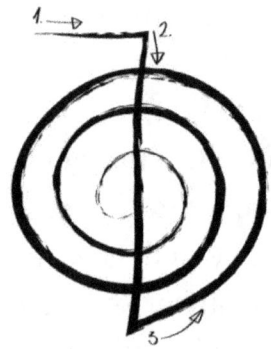

Modern (disperses, expands, gives strength to here)

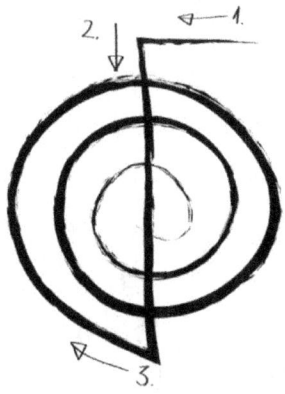

Traditional (concentrates, compresses, increases the strength)

3.3. Second symbol: Sei-he-kei

Represents: emotional healing, releasing the past; breaking emotional limitations; entering harmony; connecting with the divine; achieving emotional harmony; relieving pain; increasing the levels of energies of love; releasing aggression; getting away from negative energies and harmful radiations; passionate experience; emotional being; it is followed by affirmation: 'I relieve the pain and fill this place with the energy of love'; it releases your entire past as you create your emotional present, relieve all 'larvae' of genetic diseases and create conditions for being in harmony, emotionally and physically.

By exploring its effect on some people, we can notice very often how people who have had emotionally complicated childhood, especially those who were abandoned by one of the parents and have had poor communication with that parent ever since, do not want to spend time with the second symbol because it opens and cleanses their painful childhood wounds. However, after passing through the first stage of difficulties, caused by the feeling of pain, these people fall in love with the second symbol and use it gladly in their new relationships, especially the emotional ones. Emotional 'larvae' which you have been collecting during you present being block your growth and opportunity to become completely involved in new situations. Due to that, you always choose new emotional relationships based on the experience you have had so far, and you form certain expectations towards the outer world thus becoming disappointed when a new situation starts evolving according to a completely different pattern. Many people hold on willingly to their existing life patterns even when they are not good for them, and they do so only because they know these patterns very well. So, you can recognize everything in these patterns in advance and you just keep on telling yourself: 'It is better to stay in a bad marriage where I know everything than to make that step forward and start a new relationship, which eventually might become equally bad for me.' Bear in mind that if you use the second symbol regularly, it will create favorable conditions for you to start moving in circles which are free from such bad relationships you have been used to. Under the influence of the second symbol, your everyday surroundings will get in harmony with your light path. And this is the reason why you should use the second symbol with joy and confidence and put it everywhere around you, because it releases your past and enables you to create new situations relevant to you. The second symbol offers freedom from ego and opens you to become aware of the deep inner happiness, because you exist only in the form of a divine creature, a conscious person. You will discover the magic of feeling love and accepting everything that you are, and the second symbol which you have employed to fill the place in which you live will radiate balance and harmony. By spending time with it daily, you are on the best path to achieve enlightenment one day.

Sei condition of embryo, opening what is hidden

he-kei achieving balance; harmonizing everything that is out of balance

The full content of this symbol consists of releasing everything that is emotional, releasing the past and karma, raising the inner source of energy of love.

Sei-he-kei

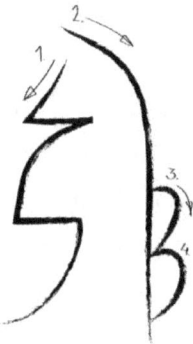

3.4. Third symbol: Hon–sha–ze–sho–nen

Represents: travelling through time and space; distant healing; determining your essential place in the world you were born; connecting with divine energies; establishing contact at a distance; opening the energy channels between us and a certain place or person; opening the path towards the karma which should be released; understanding information from any level of energy so as to become aware of an important and valuable message; opening doors to meditations; entering our inner self and our inner 'being'; entering enlightenment; the world of eternities; accepting changes as the only rule of nature; ensuring energy flows. Exploring time and space with the third symbol or travelling along the time line enables you to become aware of your optimal place of being, of your talents, people-companions who are here to support you and show you your light path towards complete enlightenment. The strength of meditation on the beam of the third symbol opens all doors so that you can discover absolute truths which support your being, thus revealing your connection to the Universal Mind and to what was given to us by the Divine. The ease of travelling along the timeline makes you aware that fear is unnecessary, because even on the day when you decide to terminate your stay on the Earth and when you change your form of being, peacefully and with lots of love towards the divine existence, and you end your life which existed in your body and unite with the Universal Mind, you will be just travelling within the general existence by changing forms.

Also, the third symbol can be used to explore our past lives. However, my personal experience is that these past lives are only past, and the parts we were supposed to become aware of are written in our mind. If, in this life, we were supposed to discover everything that had happened to us in our past lives, we probably would not be living this life. So, there is no need to explore this. Our present life path should be explored thoroughly so that we would not keep on repeating the same mistakes which lead us to deep feelings of discontent and distress. Every human limitation is created by our mind in which all our experiences have been buried not only in the form of experience but also in the form of feelings that block us, since evoking previous experience makes us feel afraid of repeating that same unpleasant emotion. The third symbol does not allow the energy from the past to become involved with the present, and especially not with the future. It puts the events in the line according to how they appeared so that we can feel the flow of energy and, consequently, in future choose emotions that we allow to occur. Our pleasant or unpleasant encounters with people can be perceived as a mirror revealing how we would behave in that situation or as a challenge to free ourselves from a feeling that we no longer need.

Hon origin; primordial beginning

sha you are shining

ze moving forward; you are on the right path

sho objective

nen silence; nirvana; peace in the essence of being

The full content can be understood as:

without past, without present, without future, only the change exists.

Hon-sha-ze-sho-nen

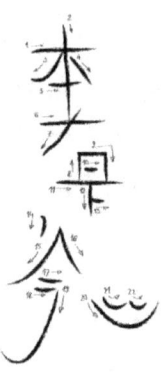

3.5. Fourth symbol: Dai–ko–myo

Represents: opening of the doors of freedom; master symbol; entering harmony; becoming united with the

Universal Mind and divine energies; surrendering ourselves in unconditional love and accepting all creatures around us; journey towards lightness; journey towards our inner selves; harmony with nature; I exist; master's gift; entering the world of opportunities; fulfilling yourself; walking freely through the physical, emotional and spiritual being. Infinity, complete unity, total support, survival without conditions; entering wholeness; absolute fulfillment of karma and unity with the Universal Mind; oneness with the divine energies.

Dai all general

ko light

myo change

Dai-ko-myo

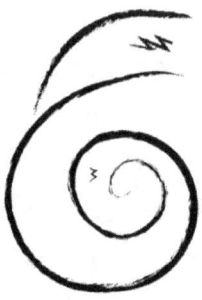

The full content brings: master's unconditional love, acceptance, understanding, support.

3.6. Fifth symbol: Raku

It reinforces the attunements of the other symbols; it opens and keeps open the energy channels along the spine; it gives a feeling of warmth which moves down your back while you are feeling how the energy is melting all your resistance, and as a result you are surrendering yourself to the light which heals you and relaxes you; the absolute, unconditional love; acceptance without exception; I am as one part of the whole I exist. You are discovering that the content of your being is complete, yet so changeable that you are just a content flowing down the river of life. You are turning into harmony and your master feels you just the way you are, open and aware of the beauty of existence and of the ease of walking through the life that is worthy of the man and their vertical evolution, which is in effect the evolution of consciousness. You are accepting your physical nature, you are releasing emotional tensions and you are travelling through your spirituality with ease.

Raku entering the lightning, balance, stability, flow;

perfect awareness of change, collector of fire; grounding.

The full content brings: only the constant flow of energy gives you awareness that the life is within you.

Raku

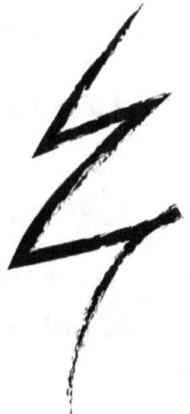

Chapter 10: The Principles And Symbols Used In Reiki

Reiki healing is founded in five basic principles. It also uses a series of symbols in order to focus mediation of the patient and the practitioner, and thus allow the energy to be channeled more efficiently. In this chapter, we will discuss the five principles upon which Reiki is based, as well as its symbols, both sacred and non-traditional.

The Five Reiki Princples

I. Just for today, I will not be angry.

Anger harbored against others, or even at oneself can create blockages in one's energy. In Reiki teaching, anger is considered the most complex inner enemy. Reiki can help to remove blockages caused by anger that may have built up in the body over an extended period of time, however it has only a limited effect on that anger which arises daily. Thus, being able to let go of anger will bring true peace of mind.

II. Just for today, I will not worry.

In contrast with anger, which comes as a result of events that have taken place in the past or are happening presently, worry deals with events in the future. Although worry is not always negative, when it becomes endless and lingers in one mind, it can bore several small holes into the body and soul. Worry requires Reiki energy to be spread throughout the body in order to heal the damage caused by it. Letting go of worry will allow the body to truly and completely heal.

III. Just for today, I will be grateful.

Gratefulness comes from the heart and grows inward. The most important element in this principle is the inner intention. Things as simple as giving thanks and forgiveness, smiling, sharing goo words and being grateful can improve your life and the lives of others and bring true happiness. Being thankful allows for the spirit to be joyful.

IV. Just for today, I will do my work honestly.

One should seek to support oneself and one's family through a respectable means, that brings no harm to others. Living an honorable life and working honestly adds abundance to the soul.

V. Just for today, I will be kind to every living thing.

Always seek to honor one's parents, teaches and elders. Being kind to others brings love into the will.

Sacred Reiki Symbols

The symbols which are sacred to Reiki healing can help you to make your personal meditation practice more clear. They can also improve your ability to channel the healing energy that is the key element of Reiki. Each sacred element affects a certain realm.

Cho Ku Rei: The Power Symbol

This is a symbol that promotes cleansing and purifying. It also protects and is associated with the physical body.

Sei Hei Ki: The Emotional Balance Symbol

This symbol represents harmony and love. It helps to balance one's emotions.

Hon Sha Ze Sho Nen: The Distance Symbol

This symbol allows for connection. It is used to perform distance healing across time or space.

Dai Ko Myo: The Master Symbol

This symbol brings mastership and empowerment when used. It can also be used to pass Reiki attunements as well as during treatments and meditation.

Non-traditional Reiki Symbols

Some of the symbols that are used by Reiki practitioners today do not come directly from the original teachings of Mikao Usui. In order to use these and learn more about their use, you will need to locate a Reiki teacher who can give attunements to the symbols in this list.

Cho Ku Rei (reversed)

This is to be used with the sacred, Cho Ku Rei when you desire to manifest something.

Tibetan Dai Ko Myo-s

This symbol is used as a substitute at ties for the original Dai Ko Myo Master symbol. Some prefer to use this to the original symbol.

Tibetan Fire Serpent

This symbol is using during the process of attunement and it stand for the Kundalini energy, or snakelike coils. These are visualized at the base of the spine, and the energy travels upward through the coils. It cleanses the chakras, and joins them as well.

Raku

This symbol is used in certain branches of Reiki in order to eliminate the gap between student and teacher following attunements.

Zonar

Zonar is believed to work across time in order to heal issues from past lives.

Harth

Used as a symbol for the heart, this symbol helps issues pertaining to love and compassion.

Halu

Halu is an amplification of the Zonar symbol, which is used for balance and love.

Antakharana

Various branches of Reiki healing use this symbol as a tool for meditation and healing.

Om

Om is a sanskrit symbol that is well known for its use in many Eastern practices, including yoga. It represents the sound of the universe and is often chanted. Some branches of Reiki use this symbol for initiations.

Chapter 11: What Are Reiki Chakras?

The different Reiki chakras are used in the practice of Reiki in order to bring focus and universal energy directly to the healer. Its purpose is to absorb all possible cosmic energy and distribute it evenly upon the body of the healer.

Clearing the different Reiki chakras is a good way to start the whole Reiki healing process. As the Reiki energy increases, the life processes from the earth to the spiritual world progresses as well, leading to a step in complete human growth. But clearing the chakras used in Reiki is dangerous if done without the proper guidance and proper supervision - if one is not fully ready to receive the chakras, a surge of energy can be overwhelming and harmful. It can lead to a possible disorientation, depravity, physical pain, and even mental breakdown.

The first Reiki Chakra is located at the base of the spine area. It helps in the body's survival, security, safety and the ability to be grounded to the earthly plane. Its physical functions are responsible for the excretion and digestion. It is responsible for the proper functioning of the small intestine and the colon, as well the sex glands, the hips, the legs, the lower back, and the rectum.

The second Reiki Chakra is found just above the genitals. It covers the individual's sexuality, self-esteem, personal power and the need to control one's emotions. It has physical influence on the ovaries, the fallopian tubes, the pelvic area, the lumbar spine, the kidneys, the bladder and the large intestines. It is also considered as the center for the body's cleansing, purification, and total health. If not attended to, it can have serious effects on the adrenal glands, leading to ulcer. It can also cause other nervous disorders and chronic fatigue.

The third Chakra is located two fingers just above the naval. When it is opened, it allows a person to function normally even when the person feels distressed. It provides the person the capability to connect, have long term relationships and can even influence into having a loving family and a happy home.

If it is abused, it can have profound effects on the sympathetic nervous system, muscular energy, heartbeat, digestion and circulation. If this chakra is blocked, the energy moving from past diaphragm will be hindered thus the energy cannot be transmitted to other parts of the body.

The fourth Chakra is located at the eight cervical vertebra of the spine opposite the heart. It allows one to sympathize with the vibrations of other astral entities so that one can instinctively understand the greater energies and atmospheres. This fourth chakra has physical influence on the thymus (located at the center of the chest behind the upper breast bone). The thymus is responsible for the proper utilization of the amino competence factor, that helps create the body's immunity to disease.

THE REIKI ENERGETIC SYSTEM

But what energetic system are the principles of a Reiki practice based on? As Reiki is a Japanese practice that was created in the early 1900s we are aware that (as with many martial arts and Ki practices that were formalized in Japan at the same time - karate, judo, aikido) the hara or tanden were considered to be the center of the body's energetic powerhouse.

The word hara literally means stomach, abdomen or belly in Japanese. Energy is stored in this point of the body from where it expands throughout the whole body.

Usui Mikao's teachings focus on building the energy in the hara. From Hawayo Takata's diary notes it can be seen that she too was taught to practice in this manner. Once the system of Reiki became more westernized in the 1980s the chakra system (an energetic system from India that has been incorporated into the New Age movement) was introduced and replaced this system - the chakra system is now commonly used in the West

In traditional Japanese teachings and exercises today the hara system is still the main focus for building a person's energy. There are, in fact, two other energy centers in the body according to the Japanese energetic system. One is the head and the other is the heart. In the Japanese Art of Reiki we have called these the Three Diamonds. By linking all three areas the practitioner creates unity and balance. Most important, however, is to first develop the lower hara, as this is the body's central axis point.

Re-establishing this connection with the Original Energy through the hara will ensure good health and recovery from illness. There is always access to a reliable source of strength whenever needed.

An inner attitude results from first focusing on the hara. From this central point there is an ability to cope with everyday tasks and sudden emergencies with an ease of understanding. This allows appropriate action to be taken in a balanced and unprejudiced manner.

1. Lower hara (approximately 3 inches (8cms) below the naval)

In this center, Original Energy is stored. This is the energy you are born with, the energy that is the essence of your life and gives you your life's purpose. The Original Energy is not only the energy you receive from your parents when you are conceived but most importantly it is the energetic connection between you and the universal life force. When the singular term hara is mentioned it is the lower hara that is being discussed. This is the symbolic energetic center for Earth Ki.

2. Middle hara (at the heart centre)

The energy in this centre is connected with emotions. It is 'human' energy connected with human experience. Through this centre you learn your life's process. From childhood through to adulthood and back to being a child. When you are a child you are without experience and as you grow older you become a child with experience. This is the symbolic energetic centre for Heart Ki.

3. Upper hara (third eye area).

This is the energy connected with your spirit. When you are connected with this centre you may see colors or you might have psychic ability. It is important for you not to become unbalanced and keep yourself centered. If you can use this energy in a balanced way, you can see beyond the immediate. This is the symbolic energetic centre for Heaven Ki.

The three diamonds of Earth Ki, Heaven Ki and Heart Ki are at the foundation of the system of Reiki. They are also at the crux of many facets of Japanese culture, religion and philosophy.

A diamond is often used as an analogy of the self in Buddhism. Each and every day a practitioner polishes the diamond by performing his or her practice. This is a constant task for humans who, in this earthly realm, attract dirt: becoming muddy and tarnished. A diamond is so sharp that it can cut through almost anything humanity attaches itself to, bringing back the true essence of life as seen in the perfection of a sparkling diamond.

FIVE WAYS TO STRENGTHEN YOUR REIKI ENERGY

TECHNIQUE 1: DRY BATHING (KENYOKU HO)

Although this is by far the most complex energy 'trick' of the five, it is still relatively simple. Doing it before each Reiki session will definitely make a difference to the flow of energy.

Method:

Put your right hand on your left shoulder, breathe into your hara (i.e. the 2nd chakra - located about 5cm below your belly button), and sweep diagonally - exhaling forcefully - across the front of your body down to your right hip.

(By 'sweep', we mean brushing your hand over your body as if you were 'sweeping' dust away from your shoulder, past your hip and onto the ground.)

Put your left hand on your right shoulder, inhale into your hara, and 'sweep' - exhaling - down to your left hip.

Put your hand back on your left shoulder, inhale, and sweep your hand - exhaling - down to your right hip.

Extend your left arm out in front of your body, palm facing upwards, arm horizontal to the ground. Put your right hand on your left shoulder - inhale into your hara - and 'sweep' along your arm - exhaling - all the way past the left fingertips.

Repeat the process on your opposite side by extending your right hand palm facing upwards in front of your body (arm horizontal to the ground), placing your left hand on your right shoulder, inhaling into your hara, and sweeping along your right arm - exhaling - all the way past the right fingertips.

Extend your left arm out in front of your body, palm facing upwards, arm horizontal to the ground. Put your right hand on your left shoulder - inhale into your hara - and 'sweep' along your arm - exhaling - all the way past the left fingertips.

Let your arms hang down by the sides of your body and feel any energetic currents that may arise (most probably in your arms and hands).

Gassho (join your hands together in prayer position [namaste] in front of your chest) and give thanks.

TECHNIQUE 2: RUBBING HANDS TOGETHER

Rub your hands together vigorously for ten seconds before giving yourself or another Reiki. This will stimulate the energetic channels in your hand, thus making it easier for the Reiki energy to flow.

TECHNIQUE 3: KEEP FINGERS TOGETHER AND HANDS CUPPED

Reiki will generally flow more strongly if you keep your fingers together (although the thumb may, at times, separate from the other fingers).

Mrs Takata, the founder of Western Reiki, apparently proclaimed: 'Scattered hands, scattered energy'. She was right, although you should naturally never be dogmatic (sometimes, after all, you may in fact desire a more spread out sort of energy).

That said, 9 times out of 10 you will feel more if you keep your fingers together.

The same can also be said for keeping your hands held cupped rather than flat on the body. The reasons for this are not exactly clear, but try it if you are not already doing so. The energy almost always seems to flow better.

TECHINQUE 4: Hover above Each Hand Position before Touching the Body

A good way to get a stronger connection to each Reiki position is to hover above it with your hands before lowering them onto the body.

The trick is to wait until you get an energetic connection and only then put your hands on the body. For some reason this makes it easier to connect to the Reiki energy of each position.

TECHNIQUE 5: Keep One Hand on the Body When Changing Hand Positions

To keep the energetic connection going (and build momentum, thus strengthening it), it is a good idea not to take both hands off your body when changing positions (the same applies when you give Reiki to someone else).

Keep one hand grounded while you move the other. Then anchor the one you have moved, and move the one you had kept grounded. That way the energetic space and connection you have established is not short-circuited.

SELF-HEALING WITH REIKI

Reiki can be used to heal others. But more importantly, it can very well be used to heal your own self. There are many ways you can do so.

Every one of us has unique personal qualities. And these qualities can be improved greatly to make you a better person. You can turn these qualities into abilities and skills, which could help you greatly in life. However, we must live well and wisely. That's the only way you can lead a life of development, growth, and healing.

Try to look back in your life. How many choices have you made that turned your life around? Every decision that you do has a powerful effect to your own existence. Your decisions become a part of what you are and who you become. Not all your choices are correct. It is but human nature to make mistakes. But what's more important is for you to learn from your errors. If you are able to understand your wrongness, you are not likely to repeat the blunder.

If you are in a spot wherein your life is in a tumble because of your wrong decisions in life, Reiki can outwardly help you to correct it. Try to heal, change, and recreate your life towards the correct path. Reiki's self-healing techniques can be very beneficial for this purpose.

One good teaching of Reiki revolves around balance. Know that the whole universe exists in a balanced state. As such, all your life's difficulties have solutions. There can't be a problem without a solution. Every challenging situation has a way out. This is what the concept of universal balance implies.

In order to find the solution, it is very important that you have the definiteness of purpose. Sustain your will and purpose. Over time, good things will happen to you. Having a definite purpose always produces the best results. Set your goals and purposes early on. Then focus on it up until you are able to attain it. Use Reiki to your advantage to further your purpose. In time, self-healing will be attained. If you pursue your purpose with passion, you will be healed faster.

Keep in mind that the mind acts similar to a magnet. It attracts everything that you think of. Think hard about your goal. And the attraction would compound greatly.

Set your mind towards your objectives. This is very helpful in improving yourself or any of your qualities. Hold the thought, believe in it definitely, and know that it will happen. Sooner or later, it will. The power of Reiki is based on this fact.

Remember that everyone has their own purpose in life. Therefore, everybody has a task to accomplish. And those tasks may require one or more special abilities. This is why you need to heal and improve yourself so that your personal qualities will be honed to perfection. It is part of your task to fully express your talents to the whole world. The Divine Being gave these talents to you. You are supposed to use them for everybody's benefits.

Chapter 12: Reiki Hand Positions And Self-Healing

Reiki self-healing is a method by which you can use this proven technique on yourself to bring the healing powers of Ki for improved energy movement and to eliminate energy blockages within your system. In Reiki, you can be your own healer. Self-healing Reiki is simple to practice daily at home. Of course, it is important that you get attuned by a Reiki Master before trying these self-healing techniques using hand placements

First, identify a quiet place where you know you will not be disturbed. Create a relaxing atmosphere by:

- Turning off or dimming the lights
- Lighting a scented candle
- Playing some soft, soothing music in the background

Sit comfortably and use the following hand positions. It is a good idea to first center yourself by using the Kanji hand positions, which include:

Kanji Hand Position #1

You can center yourself either in the sitting or standing position. Bring your hands together in front of you. Let the tips of the index fingers of both your hands touch each other while the rest of the fingers are interlaced with each other. Close your eyes for a while as you focus on your Reiki point, which is approximately 2 inches above the navel.

Kanji Hand Position #2

In this position, the tips of your middle fingers are touching each other, and all the fingers are intertwined. Hold this position for about a minute and visualize your Reiki point being engulfed with white healing light.

Kanji Hand Position #3

In this position, all your fingers are intertwined. Hold it for about a minute and visualize the energy flowing freely right through your body.

Here the 12 basic hand positions that you can use on yourself and leverage the power of Ki. You can either sit down or lie down in a comfortable position to perform the 'hand laying' techniques on yourself. If you chose to lie down, then place a pillow under your knees, and cover yourself with a light blanket if you feel cold.

Then, turn your attention inward, and focus on each part of your body right from the top of your head up to the tips of your toes. As you focus on each section of your body, pay attention to the following elements:

- What are the sensations you are feeling?
- Are you feeling tense?
- If yes, can you release the tension?

- Is there pain?
- Can you feel the pain without desiring to change it?
- Can you accept being 'in the moment?'

As you self-question in this way, you will notice tension and pain being dissolved, and you will feel an experience of being 'in the moment.' With this centering process completed, you are ready for Reiki healing.

Hand Position #1 – **Cover your face with both your hands in such a way that the fingers are cupped over your eyes and your palms are on your cheeks. The fingertips will touch your forehead when you hold your hands to your face in this manner. Remember to be gentle with your eyes and ensure you don't press or cover your nose so tightly that you have difficulty in breathing.**

Hand Position #2 – **The crown chakra is on the top of your head. For this Reiki hand position, your hands must meet at the crown chakra. Bring your hands together over your head and place them on either side** of your head to touch the crown chakra (the fingers must touch at this point).

Hand Position #3 – Touch the back of your head with one hand, and just above the nape of your neck with the other hand.

Hand Position #4 – How would you sit with your hands cupping your jaws, especially when you are angry or bored? That is the position for this Reiki hand technique. Your chin should rest in the cup formed by your wrists meeting under it.

Hand Position #5 – Hold your throat gently with one hand (similarly to holding a glass). Place the other hand between your heart and your collarbone.

Hand Position #6 – Place both your hands under your breasts when your elbows bent. Ensure your hands and elbows are comfortable.

Hand Position #7 – Place both your hands on your stomach region, which is the solar plexus area. The fingers must be in contact with each other.

Hand Position #8 – Next, move downwards, and place your hands on the pelvic bones again making sure your fingers are touching.

Hand Position #9 – Try and touch your shoulder bones at the back. If you find this position uncomfortable, then all you need to do is to put your hands on top of your shoulders.

Hand Position #10 – Bend your elbows and reach your hands behind to touch the middle area of your back. This position is for your midback.

Hand Position #11 – This is for your lower back. Bend your elbows and reach your hands behind to touch your lower back region.

Hand Position #12 – The 12th position is for your sacral region. Bend your elbows again and reach your hands behind to touch the area of your sacrum.

Hand Position #13 – This and the next few positions are best done in a sitting position lest you lose balance and fall. Hold your right foot with both your hands.

Hand Position #14 – Now, hold your left foot with both your hands

Hand Position #15 – Now, hold your left foot with your left hand, and your right foot with your right hand.

Hand Position #16 – Now, hold your right foot with your left hand, and your left foot with your right hand.

You can spend about 5 minutes at each position. Relax and feel the energy in that position. The process of self-healing in Reiki is simple and straightforward. When you have been attuned by a Reiki master, your heart and palm chakras are prepared to absorb energy from the universal life energy or Ki and transfer it for healing and health purposes.

If you have a problem reaching to your feet to hold them in your hands (Hand position # 13 to 16), then you can aim your hands to your feet and focus on the energy. The most important thing about Reiki techniques is that you have to be comfortable in the position.

Chapter 13: Verdict - Reiki Attunements/Initiations

You just require one Attunement each Reiki degree, some individuals obtain several attunements in their life times to bring added advantages that attunements deal. It is stated that numerous attunements within a certain Reiki degree puts extra worth to that degree although it is not required. The advantages of extra attunements consist of the improvement of the Reiki power that networks, fortifying of that power, recovering the receivers possess issues, quality of mind, a boost of psychic recognition, as well as increased degree of awareness.

Reiki attunements begin primarily as a cleaning procedure that impacts the physical body, mind as well as feelings. This is to obtain any sort of extra advantages that a Reiki Attunement could supply the recipient.

In the event, the Reiki master utilizes signs and also motions in a specific means to equip the recipient. The event of attunement develops a power pattern around the individual being hip to. The attunement is irreversible just if the Master utilizes the sign for the subconscious in the event.

In an attunement event the Reiki Master does the following:

They will certainly additionally advise the recipient to be open to all the encounter of attunement. At this factor the Master will certainly stand in front of the recipient as well as increase his or her hands. There could be even more compared to one recipient obtaining an attunement.

The Master will certainly stroll around the recipient one complete circle and also after that behind them. One done in front of the recipient as well as one done behind the recipient.

3. The master holds his/her left hand close to the receivers head. The left hand normally gets power while the ideal offers power.

4. With their right-hand man, they attract the sign over royalty of the receivers head. When finished with the back of the recipient the Master action's to the front

The master takes the receivers hand for a minute when they stand in front of them. He or she attracts the sign on the recipient's hand.

6. The Reiki Master after that envisions the master sign in light (some usage violet) and also gently impacts two times from the base chakra to royalty chakra. They after that gently touch the individuals 3rd eye gently, the temple.

7. Signs are after that attracted over the 3rd eye, every one as soon as well as shouting the name 3 times.

8. They carefully divide the receivers hands

9. The Master once more envisions the Master sign and also strikes from the base to royalty.

They after that Picture the master sign in their best hand and also hold it over the receivers left. The master gently puts it right into the appropriate hand, like they are marking it.

11. The Master after that envisions the master sign once again as well as delicately impacts in the location in between the receivers hands and also brings the receivers hands with each other.

12. As the Master returns the receivers restore they delicately touch the receivers heart location, envisioning that the master

is providing the recipient back to themselves.

13. The master goes back to recognize the recently hip to recipient by bowing.

14. The master once more strolls in a circle the recipient winding up before them.

Reiki attunement is the procedure by which a Reiki master passes on the power of Reiki to the Pupil so they could recover themselves and also others. The function of the attunement is to permit one to find out Reiki in order to exercise it or have the individual encounter Reiki on one more degree besides therapies.

The attunement procedure makes it possible for the one being attuned to completely open their being to the Universal Life Pressure Energies on physical, psychological, psychological, psychic, and also spiritual degrees. Every attunement one obtains opens up the recipient to greater degrees of devoutness and also recovery. Attunements, which are official initiations, are provided by a Reiki Master on 3 various degrees.

Reiki attunements are emotionally effective encounters. The attunement powers are funnelled from the Master/teacher to the pupil. Individuals that have actually gone through attunement have actually been claimed to really feel points like the 3rd eye position and also being swamped with a power they could not share.

Individuals that want to obtain hip to often get ready for an attunement as complies with (It isn't really required its recommended):.

1. No meat, fish or chicken before the attunement.

2. Not eating on water and/or juice one to 3 days prior to an attunement.

3. Lessen or get rid of caffeine prior to as much as 3 days in the past.

4. No liquor approximately 3 days in the past.

5. If you smoke, do so minimally if you could not quit totally.

6. Attempt to make use of some kind of arbitration for regarding a week in the past. It could be of your working with exactly how when.

7. Attempt to decrease viewing tv, the radio and also reviewing the information for 1 to 3 days in the past.

8. Do workout, attempt as well as stroll in nature like the park if you can.

9. Attempt as well as launch your feelings like rage, anxiety, hate and also envy in advance.

Bear in mind when you get a Reiki attunement you turn into one of a team of individuals that currently are right here to assist recover the planet. Reiki is not a religious beliefs it is a spiritual method.

Reiki degree one as well as the degree one attunement mostly profits the physical body and also opens it up in order to be able to carry the Reiki power. In Reiki degree one the record of Reiki is shown as well as the hand placements. Degree one is the structure of all Reiki as well as must be understood prior to an individual relocates on to the following degree of method.

Degree 2 Reiki and also Attunement advantages the refined physical body. In this degree the attunement offers a greater degree of power resonances in the pupil. You should have degree one attunement initially to be a degree 2 Reiki pupil.

Today Reiki is educated all over. It is suggested that time gap in between degrees in order to incorporate both experience and also exercise right into the usage of Reiki. Some pupils take years to obtain from degree one to the Master degree.

Reiki attunement is the procedure by which a Reiki master passes on the power of Reiki to the Pupil so they could recover themselves as well as others. You just require one Attunement each Reiki degree, some individuals get numerous attunements in their life times to bring extra advantages that attunements deal. Reiki degree one and also the degree one attunement mostly profits the physical body and also opens it up in order to be able to direct the Reiki power. In Reiki degree one the past history of Reiki is shown as well as the hand placements. You have to have degree one attunement initially to be a degree 2 Reiki pupil.

Degree 3 is Reiki Master. In this degree the Reiki professional obtains their last attunement and also is able to currently attune others. In degree 3 the pupil recognizes the concept behind Reiki in enhancement to the various other points.

Chapter 14: How Reiki Works

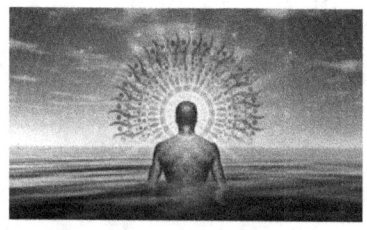

Everyone is born with a force that is specifically given to them by the breather life. This force connects all living things because they can transfer the energies from one person to another in the healing process. The human body has millions of cells, and each cell in the human body is filled with wisdom and the energy that is everywhere at the same time that they can use to heal themselves and others. The omnipresent wisdom composition in the cells of the living things provides high connectivity between them. It is part of our genetics. It runs in all our cells and cannot be separated from them, but it can only be weakened by various things.

Reiki works harmoniously. For it to work, the entire mind, the body, and the soul should be at peace. They should be balanced in that they can correspond with each other. When one's mind, body, and soul are at peace with each other, the functioning of the body and its healing are enhanced. The body will be in a position to heal itself because of biological intelligence. The cells of the body notice the balance initiated by the harmony of the mind and spirit and they can function very well and heal the body.

The flow of the life force in the body is controlled by different points. These points channel the force that the practitioner is using to the respective desired place. If it is channeled to heal the physical part of a human being, then the point's main work is to ensure that those physical parts of the human body receive this force to be healed. If the force is aimed at emotional healing, theses controlling points make sure that the force exerted is taken to the aimed place. These controlling points are called the chakras.

The chakras are like the wheels that spin the energy in the body. The primary chakras are seven, but they have others so many smaller ones that are attached to specific parts of the human body. Each chakra has its specific job of supplying energy to different specific parts of the body. They work as the energy conductors with their specific frequency attached to them. They cannot confuse and take this energy elsewhere. Just like in the case of blood vessels. Each blood vessel has its specific job that must be delivered, but the whole blood vessel's ultimate goal is to ensure that all the blood in the body is flowing well and the body is strong and healthy. Failure to which, the body system will weaken. This is the same as the chakras. Every chakra must perform its duty, and it should be delivered to the specific place, but the ultimate goal of all the chakras is to make sure there is energy flow in the whole body for it to be healed or to heal someone.

Just the same way when the blood vessels blockage causes health problems to the body, chakras do the same too. When the chakras are blocked, the body becomes weak and sick. The flow of energy in the body is reduced and at times, diluted. Due to the lack of the positive charge of the energy in the body, the energy cannot flow to the desired places because the functionality of the body is disturbed. The cells that host the energy are weak, and therefore, they cannot function properly. The energy within them is diluted. When energy flows too fast or too slow through the chakra, this means this chakra is unbalanced, and something is causing its blockage that needs to be attended to.

Reiki treatment must be full so that it can open the blockages caused by various things and rebalance the flow of the universal force within the body. The body's immune system will be fully stimulated, and the energy flow will be boosted if a person finishes a full dosage of Reiki treatment. The body will clean all the poisonous properties in it to allow the flow of the universal force. The poisons from drugs, tobacco, lack of sleep, stress, alcohol, negative habits, and so many other things will be cleaned during the Reiki treatment to make sure that the natural healing abilities are boosted to allow the energy into the body and to allow the flow to be smooth which allows the healing process to begin. A full dosage of Reiki is four days for energy flow boosting.

Different things cause blockage of chakras. It can be due to the physical body's exposure to stress or other emotional stresses and imbalances. Understanding the function of each chakra and its location can help open and energize each of the chakras to work well and be able to control the flow of energy without any problem. Different cultures around the globe have come up with ways that can be used in the stimulation of ki energy. There are ways like Tai Chi, Yoga, Meditation, but Reiki is very simple to learn and to use in the healing practice. It is not complicated.

Reiki's techniques are very simple to understand, and the results of knowing and mastering Reiki are so good and amazing. Everyone has Reiki in their bodies, and anyone can use this non-physical healing energy, however, if one is not committed to this universal life force, he may not be able to use it wholly but may only use 10% or 20% of its healing quantity. Reiki is used when hands are placed on your body or the other person's body. The energy is transferred from the hands to the hurting place because of the connection with the universal life force. The gift of Reiki has a lot of wisdom in it and unconditional love that if Reiki is used in a negative way to bring harm to yourself or others or to serve any destructive agenda, one can be able to lose it otherwise if used for the right purpose; Reiki will leave the human body when one dies. Because of its purity in love and wisdom, it likes being treated with the respect it deserves for it not to leave. The seven chakra points transmit the energy to the specific requirements a place, and these are;

The Crown Chakra

This chakra is always on top of the head. Like a crown on a queen's head, the chakra is a crown on a patient's head. This chakra is full of consciousness. The chakra is in violet or white. This chakra moves downwards up to the eyes then goes upwards again. This energy moves from the pineal glands to the upper brains, and then it continues up to the right eye. It has three main aims. It gives spiritual vision. This chakra is a dream of so many spiritual warriors. The spiritual warriors need visions to be able to know where they are moving to. This chakra also enlightens you. It opens your eyes to things you did not know. It opens your eyes and feelings to the power within you that you did not know it resides there. The intuition of things in you is all the work of this chakra. It makes sure that you understand the things that are within you and things about others.

The Third Eye Chakra

This chakra is marked by an indigo color. The position of the chakra, unlike the crown it is in the middle of your eyebrows or the forehead, and then it moves to your nose and then slightly above the eyebrows. This chakra opens up your mind and allows it to see beyond the material world. Your perception of things changes because of this chakra. How your thoughts function changes. The force in your changes and is channeled to the direct direction because this chakra makes sure of the direction — your sense of perception of things changes. How you perceive the force within you changes positively. You can tell me what to do and at what time. The energy in this chakra is sent to the spine which has very high sensitivity and then it is sent to the left eye, the lower brain, from here the energy flows to the ears and the eyes then it lastly goes up to the nervous system of the body.

The Throat Chakra

The light blue color is an accompaniment to this chakra. The throat chakra is located in the middle of the neck. Right at the center. It moves down to the center of your heart, and then it goes up again up to the center of your eyes. This chakra makes all the personal truths are heard and attended to. This chakra gives a representation of the self-expression. One is able and should express themselves differently. When they are angry, they should express themselves, and when they are sad and devastated, they should their expressions should be known. Their emotions should be well seen and attended to. All their feelings should be attended to and the only chakra to represent all this is the throat chakra. It is like a voice to expressions and the emotions of the humans.

People can communicate how they feel or what they want to do because of this chakra. The energy in this chakra allows one be able to communicate to others around him and the world at large how they feel, what their ideas are, their problems, the solutions if they have found any and they are also able to communicate to others about the progress of their healing or how to treat them. The creativity of what to be done in case of problems is handled by the throat chakra. How one creates solutions or ideas are all the energies from the throat chakra. The throat chakra is very important because it gives voice to the deepest feelings of a person.

The Heart Chakra

This chakra is represented by the rose and green colors. This chakra is located in the middle of the chest. Here all your compassion, love, and kindness come into being. The love for yourself and love for others are empowered by this chakra. The universal force in this chakra targets to bringing out the compassion for you and others. How you are devoted to the people you love or care about is brought to life by this chakra. This chakra also shows how far you have come in your spirituality. It shows the progress of your spirituality if it has gone up or reduced. The kindness you show to others is also represented by this chakra. How kind you are to people is the force channeled by this chakra to you. The energy in this chakra travels to the heart because that is where the compassion and love come from then it takes its course to the thymus gland. From this gland, this energy goes up to the lungs and the liver and finally, it rests in the circulation system.

The Solar Plexus Chakra

It has a yellow color. This chakra starts just in your belly button then it moves up to your breast bone. It is a representation of the center of the body. This chakra gives birth to all the personal powers. The identity of different things is revealed, and self-confidence is gained. The foods taken in by the body are digested, and the energies from the food are channeled to different parts of the body like the liver, stomach, gall bladder, pancreas, and the emotions.

The Sacral Chakra

The orange color is its representative color. This chakra is located below the belly button. These chakras are the master of creativity that enriches human life. It gives you the creative life that makes your; life on earthy worthy and better to live. Your chakra allows you to engage in activities that give you a lot of pleasure like good food, sex, swimming, intimacy, and so many other things that make your life enjoyable on this earth. The energy in this chakra is sent to the legs, the reproductive system, and the sensory glands.

The Root Chakra

This chakras color is red. The chakra is in the middle of your genitalia. This chakra gives all your energy a connection with earth then this energy gives you the things you need for your stay on this earth. The chakra is a great representative of life itself. The birth of all living things and how they were created are all the representations of these chakras. The energy in this chakra goes to the spine; then it moves to the kidneys, the bladder and lastly, it settles to the glands.

Chapter 15: Improve Your Physical Health

Stress and Relaxation

The most obvious, instantaneous, and dramatic benefit of reiki is its ability to decrease stress and increase relaxation. This is because reiki was actually discovered and designed for the express purpose of turning on your body's switch for relaxation. The reason it is so effective at doing so is because your body naturally wants to heal itself, and so using reiki activates that skill inside of yourself.

In today's technologically advanced, always connected, constantly trying to be more efficient, more effective, and more productive than ever world that we live in, the number of manifestations that stress takes on the body is astronomical. So for most people, this simple benefit is the most life-changing and rewarding aspect of performing reiki. Be helping to eliminate the negative energy in and around you, there becomes a concentrated amount of only positive energy in order to heal your nervous system, decrease your heart rate, and increase your dopamine levels.

The way this works is by helping you to become one with the highest vibration of your energy, which balances your chakras and various centers, which puts your entire being into alignment. It does so by allowing your energy to flow freely without restrictions, being encumbered, or reroutes. It is like if you are driving down the street and there is a detour: you are going to have to use more fuel in order to follow the new path, rather than your original one. Blockages of your chakras make your life energy do the same thing.

While we may experience benefits from always being technologically connected, it also means we are being stimulated at all times, sometimes even while we sleep! This can, and often does--even without you knowing--lead to sensory overload, which is a completely exhausting experience. It triggers the most basic, animal survival instincts that you have, and it tells you that you are under attack. And if you think about it, you sort of are! Because you believe you are now in survival mode, it activates lots of responses in your body, brain, and energy that just are not necessary for your average day-to-day life.

When you are in fight, flight, or freeze mode, your body goes into autopilot. Your heart starts beating faster, breathing becomes more labored, restricted, and shallow, your muscles start to tense up, your body temperature rises, making you sweat, and your adrenaline starts pumping. While all of that turns on, many of your bodies other functions actually shut down or slow to a crawl, because they are less crucial to your absolute survival in the moment. And all of this just because you got a notification on your phone! While these responses are necessary and important in the event of emergencies, to have extended periods of time living in this state is unhealthy and takes its toll.

Imagine all the energy your body expends reacting physiologically to that kind of stimuli, and then multiply it by the number of times you hear an alerting kind of sound--your phone notifications, breaking news, car horns, even your alarm clock. That is a lot of energy directed outside of your central flow of chakras, and away from a balanced self.

Using reiki to alleviate stress is the lifeblood of the art of healing, putting the nervous system back into a state of normal functioning, allowing all the parts of your body and energy to reset to their original, unencumbered purpose. This slows your heart rate, slows your breathing, and allows your lungs to fill more expansively, providing more oxygen for your blood stream, turning off your adrenaline, and releasing your clenched muscles.

Often times, stress will manifest itself in certain areas of the body, so some helpful areas of note include: the forehead where we furrow our brow, the stomach where we get knots, the neck and upper back where we scrunch our shoulders up, and the ribs where we hold our breath. Focusing our reiki energy to these areas will not only help to alleviate the stress we are holding in our body, but it also helps to untangle the energy blockages that happen in these areas, as well as making a mind, body, energy connection with these areas, which help us to recognize these symptoms in the future, creating a level of consciousness that we will be able to more quickly address.

Reiki's success in assisting with relaxation and stress reduction is so pronounced that many hospitals even include it in their services. The art of healing by laying of hands is that special extra care that health professionals can use to increase recovery rates and maximize patient appreciation.

Anxiety and Depression

It is not just basic levels of general or acute stress that reiki has been proven to assist with. It is also a complimentary service to treat more intense feelings of anxiety and depression. Of course, with more serious cases, reiki should not be used as the only form of treatment, but many doctors suggest using reiki in conjunction with their other forms of healing regimen.

While anxiety is a form of and a result of stress, it is different in quite a few ways. It often manifests itself in the form of sleeplessness, being irritable, irregular heartbeat, chest tightness, sudden feelings of fear, nausea, feeling out of control of their emotions, and headaches. The thing that classifies it as anxiety is its recurrence on a frequent basis that allows it to disrupt your regular life.

As we discussed in earlier chapters, reiki is especially important in helping to eliminate worry. While worry and anxiety are different things, they are related, and therefore reiki will be a logical solution to the more elevated, exaggerated, and overwhelming version of anxiety. Keep in mind the second rule of reiki, "Today only, I will not worry." Worrying is a mindset that you can control, and although it may seem automatic, that is only because you have not yet mastered the ability to stop yourself short and redirect your thoughts. Much like worry, anxiety is your mind and body telling you that something is not right and that you want something to change. While you may not know exactly why or what it is that is causing your anxiety, you do not need the source in order to treat it with reiki. In fact, the simple solution is to take action by using reiki! Something needs to change, and it could be something as simple as focusing on your energy. That is a change! You do not need to try to push the anxiety out of your mind, as this will only make it stronger and more powerful because it gets to live in the shadows and mystery. Instead, you can simply redirect your thought from how overwhelmed you are feeling to allowing your own energy to wrap around, through, over, and under those anxieties and let them melt away. This may take some practice before it becomes an automatic trigger, but over time it will become easier and more automatic.

Depression is a deep feeling of sadness, loss of interest in your regular activities, and a general sense of hopelessness. It can be acute and brought on by a specific experience and last for a relatively short amount of time, or it could also be an ongoing chronic form that follows you through most of your life. This is not simply a bad attitude or wrong mindset. Depression is a very real, serious, common, and treatable condition that actually changes the way your brain actually works.

As discussed in chapter five, reiki has many benefits to our mental health, which is why it is so successful in helping to relieve anxiety and depression. The flowing of energy does not just work on a superficial level, but rather on a deep level within your internal mood. By clearing your energy blockages throughout your body, it will help to release any stored up negative energy that could not escape before. It also brings positive energy in its place, helping you to heal yourself emotionally. This will bring yourself back to your Universal source center within your body, it aligns your chakras, which allows your heart and soul to flow freely to all parts of your body and mind. It lets your natural love seep into your whole self, as well as radiating outward to others and all the world's beings.

Giving yourself the love that has been restricted or lacking will help break the illusory patterns that have tricked you into thinking that you do not deserve the love or positive energy that you or the world has for you. When you are able to reignite that loving energy within yourself, it will also allow that same energy to come through you from the outside world.

Studies have shown that reiki has offered benefits for many aspects of treating anxiety. It has been shown to lower people's stress levels, increase relaxation, improve mood, and assist with sleep quality. Research has determined that women especially found a decrease in anxiety in comparison to those who did not use reiki. They also found that it works especially effectively for older adults for both anxiety and depression.

Physical Pain and Illness

Perhaps the most astounding effect reiki can have is on physical pain and illness. Because this art is not fully understood scientifically at this point in time, many people are skeptical of its viability. However, its results have been proven and speak for themselves. Beyond just clearing our soul and mental health, reiki absolutely can help physical manifestations of our pain and illnesses. It is about reminding your body that it has the energy to heal itself, so when you follow that logic, it actually makes perfect sense that it assists in the physiological presentation of symptoms. The amazing thing about reiki is that it does not require that you--or anyone else--understand or believe in it for it to work.

The list of ailments that reiki has helped with is endless, but includes:

Joint pain

Muscle pain

Chronic pain

Migraines

Nausea

Fatigue

Infertility

Digestive issues

Irritable bowel syndrome

Crohn's Disease

Heart disease

Cancer

Of course, just like with anxiety and depression, reiki should not be used alone as the sole source of treatment for any physical ailments, but it has been proven to help compliment other medical treatments in all sorts of cases. That being said, the reason it is so successful in complementing Western medical practices is because it is a more well-rounded and holistic approach. Rather than just addressing the physical manifestation of the pain, reiki focuses on the energy of and surrounding that issue. That pain you have been experiencing does not only live in that exact spot. Your entire body has been affected by it, and the energy in and around it has been blocked restricted, and changed because of it. In the same way that neurons transmit messages from your body to your brain, reiki transmits that same information, but on a grander and more soulful level. So if you have not treated the energy around the pain, it is more likely to linger or return.

Many people arrive at reiki to manage pain as a last ditch effort after every medical and drug solution has failed. However, it has been shown to be most effective in conjunction with traditional treatments, including physical therapy, chiropractors, massage therapy, exercise, and acupuncture, among others. By allowing the energy in your body to flow unencumbered throughout all parts of you, this will help to heal all elements of your body that need it. Putting yourself in a healing mindset allows your muscles to relax and release the tension they are holding onto, allowing for free range of motion in joints, increased oxygen flow, and sending messages to your brain that the area is becoming free of impediments.

The best part of all of it is that there are no negative side effects attributed to the use of reiki! Because the Universal life force is all-knowing, your body will only take in what it can accept, and therefore the Universe will never give more than you can handle. There will be no alternative pains or overdosing associated with reiki as a pain management treatment. In order to do so, the practitioner will use a few different techniques in order to maximize the effectiveness of the session, such as clearing out negative energy, infusing the area with positive energy, centering you within the Universe, beaming healing to the areas in need, aligning your chakras, as well as smoothing out your aura. Not only does all of this encourages your own energy systems to heal themselves, but it also assists with more traditional medical treatments by preparing your body for their treatments, making those even more effective.

Because physical manifestation of pain, injury, disease, and illness is reflective of the energy happening in your body, it only makes sense that part of healing should include cleansing and aligning the energy throughout your centers. Part of the work of reiki in relation to treating physical symptoms is focusing on the specific chakras associated with the area or source of malady. For instance, any pain or illnesses related to the lower body, addictions, and immunity issues are usually associated with the root chakra, so the reiki practitioner will transfer a lot of cleansing energy through this location. The naval chakra is tied to hip, reproductive, and low back imbalances. Most issues surrounding digestion, the liver, diabetes, or fatigue are connected to our rib cage chakra. The chest chakra affects many huge areas of concern, such as lung and breathing problems, heart problems, and breast cancer. Unsurprisingly, the throat chakra is associated with issues around jaw and throat pain, glandular issues, thyroid problems, and even scoliosis. Concerns around brain and neurological issues are linked with our eye chakra. Finally, the chakra on the top of the head is associated with exhaustion and all physical disorders that manifest themselves without a clear source.

There are countless studies that show the results of reiki are as effective as other forms of treatment. One study proved that reiki is as effective at increasing range of motion as physical therapy, improving the muscles and joints of the affected areas. Patients reported that they required less pain medication than their untreated counterparts. It also assists women who have undergone C-sections during childbirth, women who have received hysterectomies, and patients who have underdone colonoscopies in managing their pain, anxiety, blood pressure, and breathing. Many hospitals across the United States have begun including reiki as part of their treatment plans, especially for patients dealing with cancer. It is great at relieving the symptoms associated with it, especially fatigue, pain, depression, and quality of life. For this same reason, it has been shown to increase white blood cell production, improving the immune system. In fact, reiki may be more effective at reducing fatigue than even meditation!

Chapter 16: Reiki Treatments

Reiki treatment that works with energy typically falls under the energy healing umbrella. Each provides similar rebalancing and relaxation benefits. Having said this, there are differences in the theoretical foundations and how practitioners are trained. Energy healing tends to use touch techniques that require healing powers from the therapist themselves.

Therapists will then channel energy into the recipient to bring about healing. Energy healers (sometimes referred to as spiritual healers) may believe they are more vulnerable to other entities, picking up negative energy from the person they are working on.

They therefore need to carry out steps to protect themselves. Reiki healers are believed to be protected by the attunement process.

The calming effect of a Reiki treatment is also beneficial to pregnant women, supporting them on their journey. Children and even animals can benefit from Reiki as it relaxes and soothes.

Promoting a sense of well-being, many find Reiki encourages and supports positive lifestyle choices. Some even say it helps to reduce the need for alcohol and tobacco. When used in conjunction with medical treatment, rebalancing energy can help to manage symptoms of anxiety, fatigue and pain. Reiki can be used for short-term problems or in an ongoing capacity to promote overall health and well-being. Reiki is a natural treatment there are no contraindications, meaning it is generally safe to use for everyone.

You are advised however to discuss your medical history with your Reiki practitioner in case they need to take extra precautions.

Reiki treatments feel wonderful. It's as if there is a warming and healing sensation flowing through the body and the area surrounding the body. As this sensation flows through the body the person can actually feel the stress and illness leave the body.

The key to Reiki is that it treats the entire body, this includes the emotions, the mind and the spiritual portion of the body as well as the physical portion of the body. As the muscles of the body relax, the energy begins to flow freely and the person begins to feel "lifted up" and lighter. It focuses on helping the patient to relax and get in tune with their innermost being. It focuses on letting the world go and bringing in the light of peace and health.

A Reiki treatment instills peacefulness and relaxation into the person's very being. It's soothing, healing and relaxing.

A typical session of Reiki

Before you begin your treatment, your Reiki practitioner will explain to you what the treatment involves. During this consultation, they may ask you why you are seeking Reiki and details of your medical history. Providing as much detail as possible here ensures that they treat you safely and to the best of their ability. After this consultation you will be asked to sit or lie down in a comfortable position.

You do not need to remove your clothing for Reiki treatment. For comfort you may wish to remove constricting layers, shoes and/or glasses. The treatment itself involves the practitioner placing their hands gently on the body, or slightly above the body, in a predetermined sequence. The position of the hands is non-intrusive and should not cause any discomfort.

If you feel uncomfortable at any point, let your therapist know. The amount of time spent in each position will depend on the nature of your concern. The touch should be gentle and light, Reiki is not supposed to manipulate or massage.

Everyone will respond differently to Reiki treatments depending on their individual circumstances. Some people say they feel sensations during their Reiki treatments, while others do not. Some feel heat or tingling during the treatment and some report seeing colours. For some, the experience brings up an emotional response. The most common response however is a feeling of calm, relaxation and well-being.

After the treatment you may feel very relaxed, or you may feel energised. There is no right or wrong way to experience Reiki. Some people say after the treatment they encounter a 'healing reaction', like a headache or flu-like symptoms. If you are concerned about any reaction, speak to your practitioner.

Understanding Auras

For many millennia of human history, it has been a widespread belief that all objects, especially human and animal bodies, have an Aura (or electromagnetic (EM) field), and that this Aura can be visible to the trained eye. Late 19th century metaphysical science expanded on this concept with the theory that all things possess a body of etheric substance, commonly called the Ethereal Body, which is composed of the higher frequencies of subtle energy and finer pre-matter quantum particles which are intimately bound up with the physical body, as a product of creation of matter by electrofield manifestation through the quantum particles onto the physical plane.

Considering the mechanics of subtle energy fields and energy-matter interactions developed in the late 20th century academic sciences of Bioenergyinformatics and torsion field physics, and given the advanced state of modern scientific instrumentation, it seems both reasonable and logical to conclude that the Aura can be quantified and tangibly studied in an experimental manner. Indeed, since colors of light are defined by frequency, subtle energies and the bioenergy that emanates from all living things can be quantified as electromagnetic field energy that resonates with different frequencies of light.

In fact, much has been learned this century about the light properties of subtle energy fields and Auras from the works of such prominent scientists as the Polish doctor Iodko-Narkovitz, who worked with photo-electricity and electrical field measurement, the Russian inventor Semyon Davidovich Kirlian, who experimented with the qualities and meanings of Auras using photography and electrofield imaging, and the British doctor Walter J. Kilner, who eventually invented a series of goggles and filters through which anyone can see Auras in detail. Many people are also aware.

Currently the list of inventions using subtle energies as treatments and subtle energy detectors is so long that we could not possibly discuss them all.

Many scientists and doctors have been particularly intrigued by metaphysical scientists' claims that the Aura's energy-information can be used to accurately analyze a patient's psychological and emotional states. Current research further suggests that certain levels of bioelectrical Aura fields are characteristic of the physical status of the biological organism. Biological activity such as autonomic responses initiate cellular and electrochemical changes, thereby creating an environment thermodynamically favorable to the conversion of metabolic kinetic energy into electromagnetic energy.

In this process, localized bioenergy "complexes" to form a dynamic field that differentiates according to the neurological information that stimulated it. Since the skin is no barrier for such electromagnetic energy, the bioenergy field can and does radiate outside of the organism to become what we call the Aura.

The Aura is highly characterized and affected by the emotional and physical condition of a person, the biological homeostasis or imbalance of plant life, or the molecular energies inherent in and surrounding an object. This makes the reading of Auras a very useful and powerful tool for the metaphysical and clinical analysis of humans, animals, plants and objects.

The color frequencies of light of which the Aura consists are too high to be perceived by the naked eye in most cases. However, the trained practitioner can learn to perceive these frequencies naturally, by activating the Pineal Body and adjusting their brain waves to the higher frequencies of which the Aura consists.

Most psychics and metaphysical practitioners tend to see the Aura in six basic colors: red, orange, yellow, green, blue, and purple. Although the Aura itself consists of frequencies higher than those in the visible light spectrum, the electromagnetic energies in the Aura have lower, subharmonic frequencies that resonate with the frequencies of each of the colors of the visible light spectrum.

Therefore, although Auras are not visible to the naked eye, the brain may perceive the energies in resonance with certain colors, and thereby construct a quasi-visual (mental) image of seeing those colors. It is precisely in this way that humans sometimes see the Aura, and can analyze its different colors.

Seeing the Aura and interpreting its colors has been the focus of popular metaphysics for centuries, and "What color is my Aura?" is a very popular game in metaphysical and spiritual circles. However, most people "see" colors that do not match the objective frequency color of the actual Aura.

This is because they make a psychologicalassociation between the "feeling" of the Aura energy, and what the color "feels" like intuitively. The associated color is then induced magnetically into the visual center of the brain, so the person "sees" that color while looking at that part of the Aura. As a result of this common psychological phenomenon, the vast majority of literature on Auras and Aura colors are entirely subjective to the psychology of the authors, and the purported meanings of the colors are almost entirely arbitrary.

Structure of the Aura

Conclusion

While some people believe the frequencies associated with the flow of Reiki energy have been superseded by higher frequencies becoming more and more available on the planet. Even so, Reiki continues to remain a very popular and effective form of energy healing. It is safe and well documented and for a lot of people, forms their first introduction to the vast field of Alternative and Complementary healing.

Learning Reiki is a good starting point for experiencing and working with healing energy and it's a wonderful method for deepening awareness of universal healing energies in general. Reiki complements other healing methods and spiritual practices. There are no hard and fast rules about how to approach starting Reiki and Spiritual Healing.

Again, listen to your heart, and you will be guided in choosing the right experiences and the right teacher for you. Once you have learned a healing technique, to work and fun begins. To develop your understanding of, and sensitivity to Reiki, it is a good idea to devote time to regular practice.

Find a supportive teacher and practice group and pursue your continuing study. Make sure that you arrange circumstances so that you can be nurtured in your healing and growth. Keep your eyes on your goals, your mind in your heart and take things one step at a time. Love, light and healing to you on your journey. Practicing Reiki does not appear to routinely produce high-intensity electromagnetic fields from the heart or hands. Alternatively, it is possible that energy healing is stimulated by tuning into an external environmental radiation.

Reiki is an ideal complimentary therapy to go alongside other therapies. They are soothing and relaxing and may prepare the body to accept other medications better. Ideal for anyone suffering from diabetes, AIDS/HIV, high blood pressure, heart conditions and more. Reiki can work hand in hand with modern medicine and enhance the effects of modern medicine. Reiki appears to be generally safe but it should not be used to postpone seeing a healthcare professional!